ENDING THE NIGHTMARE OF POST-TRAUMATIC STRESS DISORDER

A REVOLUTIONARY APPROACH BASED ON NEW BRAIN SCIENCE

George L. Lindenfeld, Ph.D.
Diplomate in Clinical Psychology

Contents:

Contents 5

Praise 11

Who Is This Book For? 13

Foreword 15

Acknowledgements 19

Introduction, ... 21

Chapter 1   Suck It Up 25

Chapter 2   The Healing Sound 41

Chapter 3   Memory 53

Chapter 4   Emerging Therapies 65

Chapter 5   Fight, Fight, Flight or Flee 81

Chapter 6   Emerging Therapies 93

Chapter 7   Semper Fidelis 113

Chapter 8   Fidelity, Honor, Valor 131

Epilogue 147

ENDING THE NIGHTMARE OF POST-TRAUMATIC STRESS DISORDER

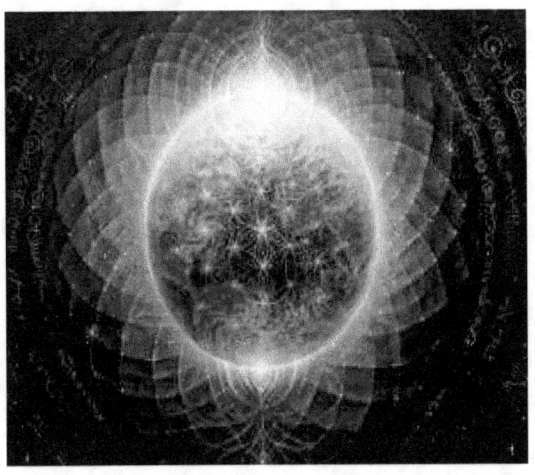

It has been said, 'time heals all wounds.' I do not agree. The wounds remain. In time, the mind, protecting its sanity, covers them with scar tissue and the pain lessens but it is never gone."

Rose Kennedy

"War is about men who love their country but even more than that, love each other. I left that battlefield knowing that they will continue to sacrifice for me. There are some events that are so overwhelming you can't simply be a witness. You can't be above it you can't be neutral you can't be untouched by it. You see it you live it you experience it and it will be with you all of your days."

Joseph "Joe" Galloway

Praise:

Shawn O'Hara – "It really altered! Afterwards, Dr. Lindenfeld said my brain had reset. As I tried to think of it immediately after, there were fewer details and the images were fuzzy where before they had been so focused. I was asked to compare the intensity from when we first started to how I was at the end of it and honestly, I said that it went from a 10 to a 1.

I still don't really understand how this happened but with one treatment, my wife says I'm a changed man. I asked her what she meant and she said, when you came home you've become that boy I fell in love with 25 years ago.

I can feel the change in me now. I laugh again. I enjoy life and I love my wife. Since my treatment, I had been able to sleep 8 hours a night like I used to with no flashbacks, no nightmares and no survivor's remorse. Also, since my treatment, I have lost 20 pounds, have more energy and I have come to enjoy life. "

Caroline Drawling - I was extremely fortunate to benefit from this new therapy before Dr. Lindenfeld's retirement. RESET Therapy saved my life or rather, gave me a life worth living after a lifetime of 'getting by' under the burden of the traumatic emotional effects of childhood incest. I can attest to the fact that

RESET Therapy is fast, to the point and it works! I sincerely share Dr. Lindenfeld's hope that many providers of therapy will care enough to learn this process and become available to help survivors of trauma live productive lives in freedom.

Dorothy Grey – "I was profoundly lucky to have found RESET Therapy. I now have a normal life after 46 years of suffering from PTSD complicated by seizures. As soon as I was upset, my cognitive functions would go haywire. People thought I was drunk. My doctor had even asked if I had an alcohol problem!

RESET Therapy leveled me out. I was able to calm myself, one trauma at a time. Even after I spent 10 years in "talk" therapy, I did not have a clear path to freedom as I have now. Something was always keeping me awake at night and triggering fears. But now, life flows and I just hit the RESET Button when I feel that something triggers an old fear. Living in peace is now possible for those of us who thought it was impossible. The reality is that it does NOT take years but happens within moments.

Who is this book for?

My intent in writing and publishing this book is to offer those veterans who continue to suffer from PTSD as well as their loved ones, the promise of hope from a member of the healing profession! I do this to replace the erroneous belief that currently pervades many of our mental health professionals about PTSD being a lifelong psychic injury that cannot be healed.

With this point of view in mind, veterans and victims of PTSD have been led to believe that they must either ingest medications designed to contain and control their minds at the expense of their personalities or, they are required to be in some form of psychotherapy for the rest of their lives, or both of the above.

This way of thinking has pervaded the civilian population to the extent that when our veterans return to either re-integrate or touch base with their families on their varied rotations, others who come in contact with them perceive that they must be careful not to trigger the veterans' inner time bombs.

It is said that PTSD keeps our warriors in a hyper-state of vigilance, but given the environment they were in and may be returning to, this state is likely necessary to protect them from harm in a dangerous part of the world. I hold a dramatically different view of the PTSD condition based on neuro-scientific research into how memory & trauma interface with each other.

My personal view is that: **although PTSD is triggered by trauma, it is really a disease of memory. The problem isn't the trauma; it's that the trauma can't be forgotten!**

With break-through research now available, just the opposite of what the cynics and doomsayers are preaching can now be said with certainty. I dare to tell our veterans that hope is alive and that quite simply said: the 'fear switch' in your mind can be placed in the **off** position when it no longer needs to be turned **on**.

A number of you will actually experience a transformative release after only twenty minutes of actual treatment with RESET Therapy. Some will require a few additional sessions depending on the complexity of the trauma each has experienced.

Foreword:

As I have read and re-read Dr. George Lindenfeld's book, it becomes very clear to me that this psychologist has immense empathy and caring for those veterans who have sought his assistance. His case studies were so compelling that I found it quite difficult to put down a particular passage until I completed reading the emotionally-charged material.

As the co-creator of the Bio-Acoustical Device (BAUD), along with my son, T. Frank Lawlis, it is my privilege to participate in the launching of this book. Furthermore, it is a joyous experience for me to experience the implementation of my professional efforts coming to a full fruition.

The case examples also validate my observations after personally administrating the BAUD protocols to over a thousand patients who have also derived positive and permanent benefits in short periods of time. Indeed, in this way Dr. Lindenfeld and I are kindred souls. This makes it doubly exciting that he is fully able to discern the full potential and power of the BAUD.

George has shared with me his struggles to find an effective means of placing PTSD into remission over the 45 years of his professional career. Like a bulldog, he has pursued this with a vengeance ultimately leading to the development of RESET Therapy. What is most revealing about this clinician's style is his intense dedication to the truth and willingness to share his findings candidly, fully and openly.

In his Memory & Reconsolidation chapter, he brilliantly connected the work of Dr. Joseph LeDoux related to memory reconsolidation, to that of my own efforts with neuro-modulation. This was the moment in time that created a full and complete understanding of how a binaural sound could alter the emotional aspect of a traumatic memory.

With the advent of brain-imaging and new neuro-assessment tools, we can now confidently declare that the brain continues to heal itself throughout our lifetime. "Neuroplasticity" (often referred to as psycho-neuro-plasticity when applied to psychological processes) is the ability of the brain to alter its circuits through training and focused intention.

People can learn to talk and walk again after brain injury because their neuronal circuits can detour neuronal signals through different circuits to enhance functioning. RESET Therapy uses this principle to rapidly restore the brain to its former level of health.

I consider ENDING THE NIGHTMARE OF POST-TRAUMATIC STRESS DISORDER to be a bold new step through which Dr. George Lindenfeld has defined himself to be in the company of very courageous pioneers. Someone who shares his knowledge with others also identifies himself as a man who cares about others.

Thank you, George.

Dr. Frank Lawlis
Diplomate in Counseling and Clinical Psychology

Acknowledgement:

As I experience the latter years of my life, I appreciate and thank all of my teachers for helping me in my transformative process. I thank each and every one of my patients for their bravery in allowing me to explore uncertain territory in their quest for wholeness.

I thank my family, fellow veterans and all who exposed their emotional wounds to me through sharing their stories. Some special people are to be singled out for their efforts including my colleague, L Richard Bruursema, for his advice, expertise and overall support; Dr. Frank Lawlis for developing the primary treatment protocol and to his ongoing commitment to ending PTSD suffering in our veterans; Dana Russell for her editing expertise and all around assistance; my daughter, Dr. Katherine Billiot and Lana Brown, (MSW), for their first read and comprehensive recommendations. Also, my expression of gratitude to my wife Ann, who put up with me and my fixation on this project each and every day.

My profound appreciation is expressed to those of my colleagues willing to pick up the baton as we move closer to the day when we can finally set PTSD victims free of their inner demons.

Introduction:

Members of our military have been tasked with repeated tours in faraway lands, often returning with looks reminiscent of those experiencing shell shock in World War II. Furthermore, there are talks of cutting our forces back by hundreds of thousands due to fiscal issues. If this were to occur, it would place increased burden on those who continue to serve.

Unfortunately, the treatment provided to our returning veterans for the trauma they experienced is shockingly inadequate. We are on the road to losing our trust in authority and in our ability to do anything about it. Indeed, we live in troubling and uncertain times.

Our therapeutic provider community, stuck in many ways in theories developed in the 1800's, appears to have become over-whelmed with the needs of so many victims of trauma and abuse. Often, the course of treatment for one individual is thought of in the context of years of intensive therapeutic intervention, which at times necessitates hospitalization for severe and complex cases.

With the volume of demand increasing astronomically, this is simply unacceptable. In addition, diagnoses are rendered freely without consideration of the impact they will have on the future potential of the diagnosed individual. This is being done within the context of PTSD being seen as an incurable disease as opposed to a normative reaction to a chronic stress condition.

So, given the above challenges, how can someone claim to have found the magic switch that can rapidly place Post-Traumatic Stress Disorder in remission? I do make this claim having treated over 100 cases during the past few years, including both military and civilian trauma patients,

I can confidently say that all of the people I have treated who have specified trauma such as war experiences or horrendous motor vehicle accidents, remain in remission, responding to a new form of treatment quickly, and for some, immediately.

It's time to get to the heart of my claim that PTSD can rapidly be placed in remission by resetting the fear switch within the brain. Chapter One will take you right into it by illustrating the treatment of a veteran who experienced severe PTSD.

I trust that this journey will be as exciting and eye opening for you as it was for me in arriving at this time of sharing. Although this book is primarily focused on PTSD, it is my plan to write and publish other books that will build on this foundation that I'm providing for you. I have included one Complex

PTSD chapter at the request of my editor in order to let those suffering from childhood trauma also know that RESET Therapy offers a solution for them as well.

Please be assured that what you read may also apply to any other anxiety-based mental health conditions such as phobia, obsessive compulsive disorders or other fear-induced conditions. Additional Kindle offerings will focus on issues closely associated with PTSD such as depression, unresolved grief, addiction, chronic pain and complex PTSD.

I want to help you to be able to break through the current limitations that restrict you from truly experiencing a positive transformation in your life. I also know that if you're reading this text, you are among those who wish to 'break through walls' that currently constrain you from becoming the person that you are truly capable of being.

When you have experienced a complete healing of mind, body and spirit, there will be no remaining doubt in your mind that finally there is a transformative treatment that really works for PTSD and so many other conditions!

Chapter One:

'Suck It Up and Truck On'

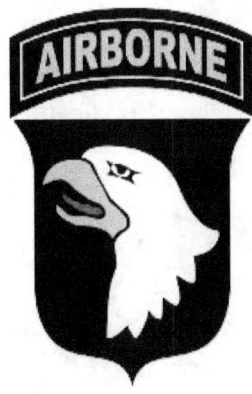

Katherine B. Therrell, NCC, LPC-S, a counselor in Asheville, North Carolina stated that: "This is the story of a modern miracle involving the interweaving of three lives, the application of science, and the awesome ability of the human brain to heal itself in response to a novel stimulus that can only be described as miraculous.

"My client Shawn came to me for counseling on September 9, 2014 for help with an anger problem. His Employee Assistance Program authorized 6 pre-approved counseling sessions to try to resolve this problem. During our initial conversation, he told me that he was currently serving in the Army Reserves. As we talked further, this army veteran revealed that he had suffered severe trauma while on military duty at a time when the military's answer to PTSD was to 'suck it up and truck on'.

"Asking for help was seen by him as a sign of weakness that was a threat to his military career. After 20 years of 'sucking it up', unresolved trauma threatened his marriage, his health, and virtually every aspect of his life.

"My initial thought was to treat him with EMDR Therapy, an evidence-based practice for trauma victims. However, I was concerned that EMDR might require more than 6 sessions. Ethically, I was torn between treating the trauma or simply trying to treat the symptoms.

"Fortunately, ten days later I attended a presentation by Doctor George Lindenfeld who claimed to have successfully resolved PTSD in soldiers using neuromodulation procedures. The methods he described were similar in theory to EMDR but went a step further. He claimed he could achieve satisfactory results often in one treatment session.

"Doctor Lindenfeld wanted to attain scientific evidence by providing a comparative fMRI treatment analysis in a PTSD case study. He hoped that this initial attempt would make it possible for a formal research project to be undertaken sometime in the future.

"When he asked if anyone knew of a veteran who might be interested in participating in his initial research, I immediately thought of my client. I talked with Doctor Lindenfeld following his presentation and we agreed that my client would be a good candidate for the study. I presented the idea to this client and he eagerly agreed.

"Shawn underwent the neuromodulation procedure on our second visit and after about 15 minutes said his body felt 'loose'. To him, the traumatic event now seemed fuzzy when he tried to recall it. On a scale of 0 to 10, with 10 being the highest level of disturbance possible and 0 being no disturbance at all, he stated that his degree of disturbance had dropped from 10 to 1. The positive changes my client experienced during the week that followed included more normal sleep patterns, more tolerance for minor annoyances, less anger and more joy in life.

"His recovery from PTSD was truly amazing. During his next and final session with Doctor Lindenfeld with me present, he reported having only one episode of night sweats in the past week. I was aware that he had been the victim of child abuse in a dysfunctional family, so I concurred with Doctor Lindenfeld's opinion that there was still something else that my client needed to process.

"Doctor Lindenfeld asked him to focus upon past disappointments while listening to the sounds. This time his countenance became sad and his body slumped as he erupted into a catharsis of tears and moans. He released years of suppressed feelings he had previously been unable to acknowledge.

"Though he may need to continue processing these feelings through counseling, acknowledging their existence was a major step in understanding his emotional pain."

Shawn's Story

"I used to be scared to talk but I want to talk now. My name is Shawn and Doctor Lindenfeld has helped me to be the person I was meant to be. Because of being 'fixed' so quickly and being skeptical about it at first, I want to reach out to help anybody I can that is suffering from PTSD. Because of this, I've given him permission to tell you my story and provide you with my name.

"I'm now a witness to the fact that other people with PTSD can be fixed as well. I was a skeptic, but I'm not one any longer. First, let me provide you with my wife's observations of the changes she has seen in me after only two treatments."

Lynn's Story

"My husband and I dated in high school. Twenty-some years later, we reconnected and married. I remembered him as being easy-going, funny and happy with my family always referring to him as 'sweet Shawn.' This made it all the more difficult to understand during our first few years of marriage why he seemed so unhappy.

"I would say to him, 'you're never happy' or 'you're so hateful, everything irritates you.' I knew something was beyond his control; something had happened in those years we were apart. I had a mental checklist of things to avoid; things I knew would turn him into the Shawn I was afraid of. Trying to avoid those triggers made life difficult.

"I would dread things like holidays, bad news, work issues, interaction with family members and typical daily problems. I would even try to remind myself not to speak while we were watching TV so as not to irritate him. I felt like Shawn had no gray area in his emotions; things were either good or as bad as they could get.

"He was a ticking time bomb living in a world of black and white. When he would have what I referred to as an episode, I knew it was coming. By 'it', I mean objects being thrown, hateful things said,

29

threats of leaving me or divorcing me resulting in the worst fights imaginable without coming to blows.

"This would be followed by Shawn hating himself for how he had just behaved and begging me to forgive him. It was confusing to feel so hurt and to also feel like Shawn did love me and honestly had no controls over his actions.

"When Shawn had the new procedure, I tried not to get my hopes up. I thought at best, maybe there would be a placebo effect. Now, many months later, I am convinced that this made a real difference.

"Shawn hasn't had an episode since having treatment. We had our first holiday in two years where everything went well and there was no typical fight. I've seen him actually laugh out loud. This seems trivial but it's not. This was once a rarity!

"I've seen the daily frustrated look erased from his face. Shawn's been able to deal with things and not go to that dark place he once knew. He has started to sleep better, has more patience and actually seems happy.

"I don't understand how the procedure worked but I know that it did. I got back that 'sweet Shawn' that I knew from high school." - Lynn

Shawn's Story (Continued)

"Once again, I'm Shawn and I was born to a single mother who didn't have much money having to work three different shifts at times to support us. So, growing up, the military really was my only option. I enlisted in the Army when I was 15 years old back in 1988 having to wait a year until I was graduated and went in at age 17.

"I attended basic training at Fort Knox, Kentucky and then went on to Advanced Individual Training at Fort Rucker, Alabama. After, I was stationed at Fort Campbell, Kentucky. In August 1991, I deployed to Iraq and upon returning I volunteered for airborne training and then was PCS (Permanently Changed Stations) to Fort Bragg, North Carolina.

"For the next several years everything was fine. I was in an airborne unit that underwent frequent airborne operations. During the next 3 to 4 years, I didn't have any accidents or mishaps occur. That's up until the morning of March 28, 1994, when trauma permanently entered my life.

"The day started out as every other day beginning with physical training, attending to personal hygiene needs and then a hearty breakfast. We were getting our equipment ready for another routine airborne operation when we loaded on the bus, like we always do, setting off to Pope Air Force Base.

"We went through a routine check at Greenramp, our loading destination. We arrived later than the other paratroopers so we were behind in everything we were needing to be doing. Then, out of nowhere, another soldier yelled, 'The pilot's punched out.'

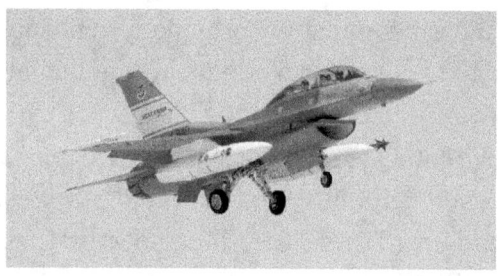

"I noticed an F-6 jet doing low approaches and also noticed that C–130s were also coming in. What crashed was an F–16 that had a midair collision with a C–130 which caused the F–16 to crash into Greenramp. After the accident, I often asked myself, why did I survive? I've replayed the accident over and over in my head and still can't understand how I got to survive and others didn't.

"When it happened, I heard the crash and looked behind me and all I saw was a wall of fire. I ran as fast as I could but it seemed to be catching up to me.

Then, someone yelled, 'over here.' I ran to that voice and dove behind a wall. When I dove, I felt the intense heat of the fire behind the wall and as I turned my shoulder and looked, I saw it go past me. I got up, came around the wall to see what happened.

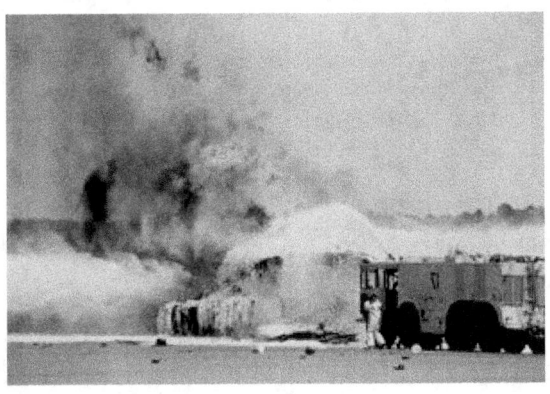

"It looked like what I imagined hell to be. There were people screaming, running and on fire. I ran to the first person that needed assistance. He was a male soldier but I couldn't tell what race. His lips were gone, nose was gone and eyes were gone. His whole body was charred and all he asked for was water. I gave him water and stayed with him until he passed.

"We helped as many people as we could by creating makeshift ambulances out of military vehicles and directing helicopters to the landing zones. After we got all the wounded and the dead out of the area, we formed up in a group and our commander had a talk with us.

"I remember I was wearing a cross around my neck. The Colonel came up to me and slapped me on my face and said, "I guess that God was watching over you." I guess he wasn't watching out for the other guys with crosses that didn't make it that day.

"We all loaded up on the empty trucks that still had blood and flesh inside of them and we went back to the motor pool. Nobody said a word and we just loaded up in our personal vehicles and went home.

"When I went home, my wife at that time said she had heard about an accident and wondered if I was there. I told her yes, I was in the middle of it and she didn't seem to be too concerned. I remember getting the bloody clothes off and throwing them in the laundry and taking a bath where I fell asleep in the tub. I woke up, dried off and went to bed and never talked about the incident from that day on.

"When the plane crash happened, we reacted like we were trained to but there was no training on what to do afterwards. After that Colonel talked to us, we never spoke of it again. The Army's attitude towards PTSD was to 'suck it up and truck on.' Several weeks after the accident, the only thing mentioned about the crash was the total number of deaths and injuries which included 24 dead and hundreds burned.

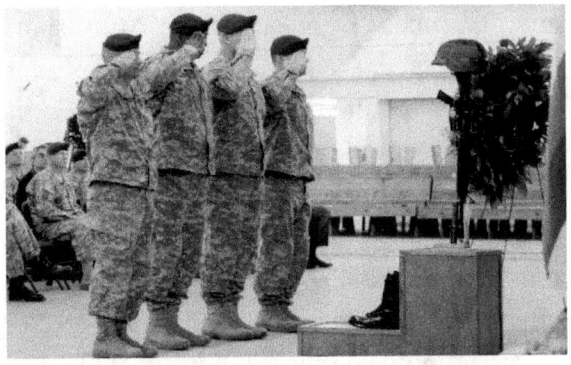

"We had a small ceremony dedicated to those who passed and a small ceremony to award the heroics done on that day. That's all that was ever mentioned of that. The other soldiers that were there never spoke of it. To this day, I don't know how they dealt with their trauma. It's been 20 years and I saw an article in the Fayetteville Observer. There was one small paragraph and that's all I ever heard of it.

"When my wife wasn't so concerned about me being in the middle of the accident, I felt like she really didn't love me that much. From that point on, our marriage took a decline. I lost interest in her and in doing anything with her. I felt that since she didn't love me, why should I love her back.

"We slowly grew apart over time and I would volunteer for every mission that came down the pike. I went on a mission where we invaded Haiti in 1996 and when I got back, she was gone and it didn't bother me that much. I got out of the Army shortly after and moved back home to Captain, North Carolina and then reunited with my wife.

"I thought that the military was the problem but in fact, it turned out to be the traumatic experience. We stayed together for about 3 years after and she wound up meeting somebody new. We filed for divorce and I didn't seem to mind so much. I didn't feel like I was losing anything.

"Looking back on it now, I know that the trauma changed me. I used to be compassionate and loving and I turned cold and callous. I used to be funny and people wanted to be around me and after, I wasn't funny like I used to be and I didn't like to be around people. After the trauma, I noticed that I didn't sleep as much. I started having nightmares. I would see the burning bodies and I didn't want to see them anymore.

"I would stay up late until I was totally exhausted and then pass out either on the couch or be woken up and told to go to bed. I figured if I didn't dream, I wouldn't have the nightmares. On one occasion, I actually hit my wife while I was asleep. While we were still together at Fort Bragg, North Carolina, I noticed the changes in myself and I couldn't figure it out.

"I tried other things to make myself feel more comfortable. I reverted to alcohol. My choice of drink was vodka and I would drink until I passed out. I was more fun while I was drunk and it seemed like my wife enjoyed being around me while I was drinking, but the drinking got to be too much.

"After I got out of the Army in 1996 my wife and I divorced 3 years later. I got remarried a year after that with this one lasting for two years. My second wife said I was an 'ass hole' because I was cold hearted. It was the same thing that I was dealing with like when I was with my first wife. I was uncompassionate, unloving and unsympathetic.

"I didn't realize it then, but the trauma had really changed me a lot. I went several years being very promiscuous and drinking a lot and going to the clubs. It started affecting my work life and my health.

"I reunited with my high school sweetheart, who I wound up marrying and I love her very much. When she said to me, you have a problem and you need to address it, I didn't want to lose her too so I looked into getting some counseling. I started counseling with my wife in late September, 2014 by meeting with Katherine and we started talking about what my problems were. I didn't realize it, but I've since come to realize that I suffered from PTSD.

"My therapist talked with me about a new, experimental treatment and I told her that I was willing to try anything. She introduced me to Doctor Lindenfeld and we three began the course of treatment for my PTSD. I really didn't believe that Doctor Lindenfeld or anyone else could possibly help me after all these years but I didn't want to lose my wife.

"My first treatment visit occurred in October, 2014. I had only slept for six hours as usual after the crash happened so I arrived anxious and hopeful at the same time. I remember having knots in my stomach and really being scared to death. I had a dream that night before the treatment and woke up soaking wet from sweat. This happened once or twice a month for me.

"When I listened to the sound through the headphones and put myself into the trauma, I swear that I was really there. I felt a cramping in my stomach and then the heat and then came the pain when I dove behind the wall. I saw all the carnage, the bodies and then it became hard for me to focus on it.

"It really altered! Afterwards, Dr. Lindenfeld said my brain had RESET. As I tried to think of it immediately after the treatment, there were fewer details and the images were fuzzy where before they had been so focused. It didn't feel as physical anymore either. I was asked to compare the intensity from when we first started to how I was at the end of it and honestly, I said that it went from a 10 to a 1.

"I still don't really understand how this happened but with one treatment, my wife says I'm a changed man. I asked her what she meant and she said, when you came home from that treatment you've become that boy I fell in love with 25 years ago. I can feel the change in me now. I laugh again. I enjoy life and I love my wife.

"Since my treatment, I had been able to sleep 8 hours a night like I used to with no flashbacks, no nightmares and no survivor's remorse. Also, since my treatment, I have lost 20 pounds, have more energy and I have come to enjoy life. I never sought counseling before because I thought it would negatively affect my military career. I wanted it this time because I didn't care what the repercussions would be. I just didn't want to lose my wife.

"Talking with my therapist and my wife, I came to realize that I was a very mean man. I would say cold things to my wife like, 'I'm going to divorce you' or,

'I wish you would die in a fire.' I never meant any of that stuff. I couldn't understand why I was saying these mean and harsh things to someone I love.

"I'm still have a hard time believing that listening to a sound for 15 minutes while I put myself in that trauma again could change my life this way. Dr. Lindenfeld said that he'd like to order a tee-shirt for me that says: "My PTSD limbic brain has been RESET." I think that's a wonderful idea!"

Chapter Two

Neuromodulation –The Healing Sound

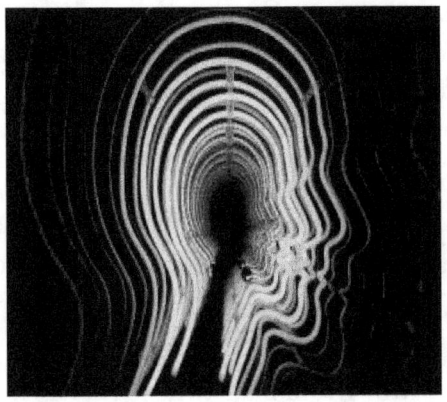

Sound has been utilized in various cultures for thousands of years as a tool for healing. For example, the drum is the oldest known instrument in the world dating back to 4000 BC in Egypt.

Among animals, Macaque monkeys drum objects in a rhythmic way to show social dominance. Other primates make drumming sounds by chest beating or hand clapping. By using rhythm and frequency the human brain can down-shift our normal state of focus and concentration to that of a meditative state.

This same concept is utilized in meditation by regulating the breath, but with sound it's the frequency that is the agent which influences the shift. Loud sounds can elevate our stress levels, create imbalances in our nervous system, lower our immunity and in extreme cases, cause hearing loss.

When we are stressed, our whole relationship to sound changes, and regular everyday sounds can become magnified and contribute to the feedback cycle of the stress, amplifying it even more.

In the realm of healing techniques, sound has been used for thousands of years yet, it's also on the frontiers of modern neuroscience.

George Gershwin wrote that, "Music sets up a certain vibration which unquestionably results in a physical reaction. Eventually the proper vibration for every person will be found and utilized."

Much of the current work on sound is based on the early 70's research of biophysicist Gerald Oster. Oster showed that when a tone is played in one ear and a slightly different tone is played in the other ear, the difference causes the brain to create a third, internal tone, called a binaural beat. What's important for you to know in this discussion is that the properly set binaural beat is the means through which we eliminate the emotional component of the PTSD condition.

Hearing is one of the most crucial means of survival in the animal world, and speech is one of the most distinctive characteristics of human development and culture. The science of acoustics spreads across many facets of human society music, medicine, warfare, architecture, industrial production, and more.

Likewise, animal species such as songbirds and frogs use sound and hearing as a key element of mating rituals or marking territories. Physicists and acoustic engineers tend to discuss sound pressure levels in terms of frequencies, partly because this is how our ears interpret sound.

What we experience as a "higher pitch" or "lower pitch" sound are pressure vibrations having a higher or lower number of cycles per second. This is also an important element in properly setting the sound levels to create a transformative platform.

Binaural beats are slightly differing sounds with each heard in one ear that are proposed to induce relaxation, meditation, creativity and other desirable mental states. This effect was discovered in 1839 by Heinrich Wilhelm Dove with greater public awareness emerging in the late 20th century.

Binaural beats can be experienced without headphones; they appear when playing two different pure tones through loudspeakers. The sound perceived is quite similar with sound events that seemingly move through the room at low-frequency differences and diffuse sound at slightly bigger frequency differences.

There have been a number of unsubstantiated claims regarding binaural beats including that they may help people memorize and learn, stop smoking, help with dieting and improve athletic performance.

The sensation of binaural beats is believed to originate in part of the brain stem which appears to be related to the brain's ability to locate the sources of sounds in three dimensions and to track moving sounds.

Interestingly, a study of aphasic subjects who had a severe stroke versus normal subjects showed that the aphasic subject could not hear the binaural beats, whereas the normal subjects could.

One hundred and thirty-four years after Dove's original discovery, Gerald Oster published, "Auditory Beats in the Brain" (*Scientific American*, 1973). In particular, Oster saw binaural beats as a powerful tool for brain research focusing on questions such as how animals locate sounds in their three-dimensional environment.

Oster also considered binaural beats to be a potentially useful medical tool. He believed that it could not only be used for finding and assessing auditory impairments, but also for more general neurological conditions because binaural beats involve different neurological pathways than ordinary auditory processing. For example, Oster found that a number of his subjects who could not perceive binaural beats suffered from Parkinson's disease.

At this point, let me introduce you to the BAUD (Bio-Acoustical Utilization Device). I use the term 'target' and suggest to my patient that we are going to turn off the 'switch' in the brain that produces the PTSD/trauma symptomology. The patient sets the lower two sound level dials of the BAUD as illustrated below with eyes closed.

At times, I will note a large difference in the lower setting and will advise the patient to have their hearing checked. Occasionally an individual with hearing loss will come in with hearing aids. I'll try the settings with them on and then off to get the best treatment option available for RESET Therapy.

Let me help you to fully understand what RESET Therapy stands for. It is the treatment process that interferes with a targeted memory being restored repeatedly after it is selectively lit up in the emotional part of the brain by the patient's intentional focus.

We next focus on the upper dials to set them to connect with the selected trauma. When the individual connects (resonates) with the trauma, I will ask them to rate it on a 0 to 10 scale with 10 being the highest. This aspect of the 'tuning in' requires much expertise to get it right so this is not a do-it-yourself' type of project.

When the sound is set correctly, a five-minute trial is initiated with inquiry made of what the patient experienced. Often, he/she will use words such as: fading, diminishing, dwindling, disappearing, becoming foggy or drifting away from the target.

When the full treatment session occurs, the patient 'runs the script' internally for a full 15 to 20 minutes. More often than not, the patient reports that his inner mind took over from the script and ran its own agenda of nightmares, flashbacks, etc.

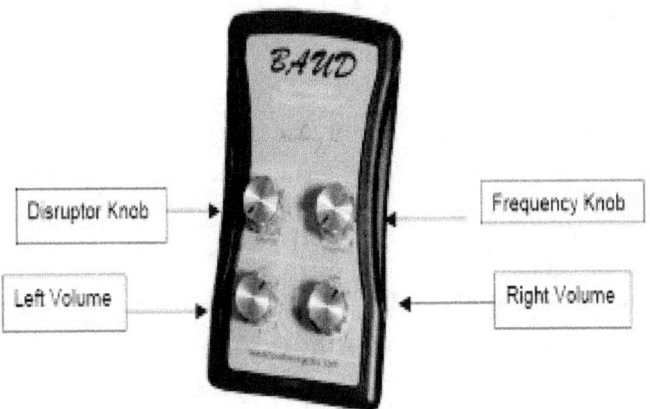

Paradoxically, after 5 minutes or so, the sound is reported by many to become increasingly comfortable. When asked after, what had occurred, the patient typically reported a sort of dissolving or fading effect of the targeted material.

When asked after the treatment to discuss the target, the patient typically says something to the effect that he can recall exactly what happened but the uncomfortable emotional component was gone. It is at this point that the patient's trauma can be conveyed verbally, fully and completely, rather than in the fragments that previously predominated.

The patient is asked to remain skeptical to the reset and is instructed to call 24 hours later to report any changes that may have occurred. Often, I will receive positive feedback about a full night's sleep, none of the previous cold sweats at night, no anger outbursts at loved ones, no horrible flashbacks.

It still gets to me at an emotional level when I hear this. I feel like I've brought someone back from the brink. When you get to experience this personally it's like nothing else you've encountered before. You begin to anticipate the excitement of what this day and the days to come will bring as you experience change through this transformative process.

This is the point that insight begins to flow to your mind and you are able to fully discuss your experiences. After the trauma switch, has been flipped, you once again have an opportunity to become the person you were before your trauma encounter. Finally, when this procedure is provided carefully by an adequately trained professional, the flashbacks and other negative sensations are gone!

I personally image the part of us that 'flares up' in the brain with PTSD as being equivalent to an angry cobra with its hood flared, ready to strike at any perceived intrusion. To be blunt, one of the veterans I've treated previously referred to it as a, 'pissed off cobra.' After the binaural sound has been properly tuned in, the cobra becomes 'defanged' and the venom neutralized. It is only at this point that discussion with the therapist can safely occur without the treatment provider being susceptible to absorbing the poison.

What incredible new treatment could possibly allow the therapist to do seemingly miraculous work while blocking the cobra's poison from doing its invasive poisoning of all who come close to it?

The secret to fending off this destructive emotional 'virus' is to have the patient 'light up' the limbic brain's circuitry internally by focusing on the emotional experience: deeply sensing it, visualizing it, experiencing it in every way possible but keeping it **INSIDE**. By the way, this is where our imaginary cobra lives in an area called the Amygdala that is part of the Limbic System of the brain.

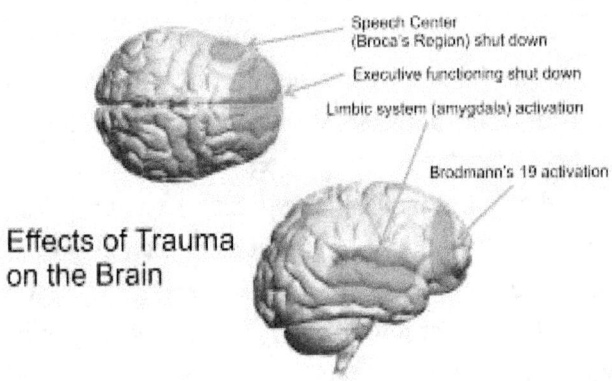

Speech Center
(Broca's Region) shut down

Executive functioning shut down

Limbic system (amygdala) activation

Brodmann's 19 activation

Effects of Trauma
on the Brain

If we looked at it through an fMRI, specific areas deep within the brain such as the Amygdala would appear to be activated (flared) and other brain areas

49

such as the speech center located in the left hemisphere would be shut down, going off line when the trauma is triggered. The area that is associated with making complex decisions in the prefrontal lobes referred to as 'executive functioning' also goes off line when the trauma is reactivated.

Perhaps this is the reason that talking to someone in the depths of their PTSD despair hardly ever does anything but frustrate the speaker whose words can't be received by the supposed listener. Also, perhaps this is why the person with PTSD seems dumfounded by tasks that he/she was previously well able to manage.

Another area located in the visual cortex (excuse me for getting a little technical here) is called Brodmann's 19. This probably sounds to you like a designated area where the federal government stores aliens from other planets. All kidding aside, this part of the brain first receives images conveyed through the eyes that rekindle visual aspects of trauma often referred to as flashbacks. Other senses such as smell, sound, visceral sensations also appear to be reactivated and seemingly newly experienced. I will consequently refer to the above pattern as the Neuronal Model of PTSD.

To reiterate, when an individual is traumatized as evidenced in fMRI studies, the following happens.

The connection to the prefrontal cortex shuts down leading to an absence of the ability to understand and a diminishment in the executive functioning that previously existed.

Secondly, the speech center located in the left hemisphere of the brain suffers the same fate with the PTSD sufferer being left with an ability to address only fragments of the trauma. This makes it difficult for him/her to fully articulate what happened in the first place. It also filters the ability to hear from others in a complete and meaningful way.

The person becomes unable to fully express what has occurred. Furthermore, he/she becomes unable to benefit from what others say. Next, the Limbic System becomes over activated perpetuating the 'fight, flight or freeze instinctual response.

The same over-activation occurs within an area called Brodmann's 19 that is part of the visual system. This is where the visual flashbacks emanate from. I'm sure there is more to it but this constellates a major part of this network.

At this point we have accomplished stage one of this incredibly effective treatment that can place PTSD into remission. Others are trying to connect with specific areas of the brain such as the Limbic System by placing electrodes in the brain through invasive surgical procedures. Contrast that with this non-invasive and safe form of intervention which is relatively free from side effects.

The treatment is called RESET Therapy (Reconsolidation Enhancement by Stimulation of Emotional Triggers), a term that I will expand upon as we discuss the next stage of this intriguing treatment. There is no question that this intervention is a form of Exposure Therapy. However, I find that it is necessary for the patient to go through this ordeal only one more time.

Let me say that again, more often than not, it is necessary for the patient to go through this ordeal only one time. After they experience rapid relief from this initial encounter, my patients tell me that they have little hesitation in engaging in the process again if a new target surfaces as often as required. This is the moment that hope and trust becomes a possibility replacing the false conviction that change is not possible.

Chapter Three:

Memory & Reconsolidation

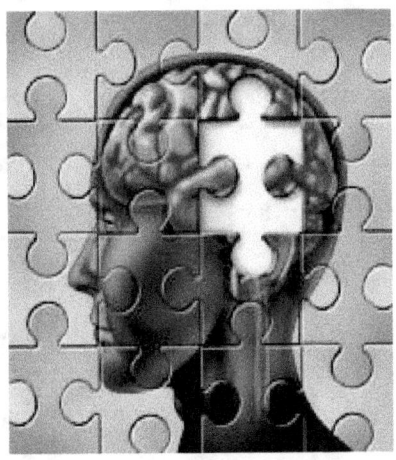

The next topic we will get into is called Memory Consolidation/Reconsolidation. Recent advances in brain imaging (PET and fMRI) have opened new doors to our understanding of PTSD and other anxiety-related disorders.

It is now known that the symptoms associated with this condition closely interweave with memory circuits in the emotional center of the brain. To describe it differently, the cobra doesn't forget! Get ready for a revelation: PTSD is really a disease of memory. The real problem is not that the trauma happened in the first place, it's that the memory of the trauma can't be forgotten.

The emotional charge that accompanies the memory remains hair-trigger and intrudes into all aspects of functioning. The charge continues to infect the patient with the cobra's poison until we are able to reset the brain circuitry thereby ridding it of the poison's ongoing effect. This is similar to turning off the light switch. I again assure you, it can really happen.

Historically, we have thought of memory as remaining constant over time. In line with the concept of permanency, it has been thought of as something etched in stone that remains unchangeable.

As society and technology advanced, a newer model of a filing cabinet in the brain was thought of wherein memories were retrieved when needed simply by 'pulling them out'. You simply attend to it and the brain finds the right cabinet and drawer and out comes the selected memory.

With the emergence of computers, the model shifted accordingly with the notion of a 'supercomputer' that provided rapid connection to stored memories within the brain's computer bank. Advances in neuroscience have helped us to understand that memory is not located in a single storage complex in the brain, but rather is a brain wide function scattered throughout the entire cortical system.

When we focus on a particular object such as an apple, each part of its essence is drawn from different regions of the brain such as the sense of taste, color, shape and then finally, how we apply meaning to it and our attraction or aversion to it. This happens so rapidly that we are unaware of the blending of this data into our conceptual understanding. We refer to this as 'retrieval' and the way it gets in there the first place is called 'Encoding'.

The Hippocampus is the recipient of these varied perceptions which then forwards them to the prefrontal cortex which analyzes the material to determine significance in regards to long-term memory storage.

So, following the apple model, if you've recently started to eat a fantastically delicious looking apple and discover that it has a big, squishy worm in it, you'll likely react differently the next time you consider biting into another deliciously looking apple.

I'll avoid getting too technical about the process that chemically converts information into electrical pulses allowing connectivity between varied cells in the brain and body. Suffice it to say that over time, with repetition, the pathways strengthen within an established network of cells extending out further and further depending on the importance given to the circuit. Constant reorganization is occurring such as the earlier discussed worm in the apple experience.

These changes strengthen with use, resulting in complex networks that can lead to improved development of skill such as a child learning to play baseball. Practice and time makes smooth the throw, strengthening the likelihood of the bat hitting the ball and increasing the probability that the child can get to first base with a hit.

To develop this ability, the child must first be able to pay attention to the task. This allows the brain to store information through a filtering process referred to as encoding. A number of different theories exist regarding how information is stored in the brain. A three-part process seems to be favored that includes sensory data first coming in through varied channels such as sight, smell, touch, etc.

The child perceives of this such as when he is holding a bat and looking for the ball that is being thrown in his direction. Next, selected material is placed in a short-term memory state. This is one of the abilities that are assessed when a neuro-psychological evaluation is conducted. He swings, likely misses the ball and then adjusts what he is doing over time to obtain the desired outcome.

We know that short-term memory is limited in its storage and hold time capacity to around seven items with a time limit being around 20 to 30 seconds as the typical duration time. Of course, memory experts can increase this dramatically by chunking the material such as what we do with telephone numbers.

A transfer process takes place from short-term to long-term storage based on a number of factors including significance of the material, repetition, emotional charge, etc. Retrieval occurs subconsciously with the material rising from that level to consciousness.

Forgetting is often a result of insufficient attending in the first place such as forgetting where you've put your keys. Next, you may not have retained where you put them because you were preoccupied with something else. And then finally, you may have difficulty with retrieving the information due to a number of other reasons such as distraction.

I'll end this discussion without going into the specifics of what occurs with the aging process. At times this results in memory deficits leading to cognitive impairment although most of us can expect adequate memory abilities through our 70's. I find that at 75 I have to put my keys, wallet and glasses in certain places. If I don't do this, the hunt begins! Now we move on to serious matters.

In 2012, T. Agren defined fear memories as being, "made stable and permanent through a process called consolidation that stretches on for hours after the initial encoding." This means that after a traumatic experience, each time a fear memory is recalled; it again becomes unstable and is restored in the brain through a process called Reconsolidation.

In other words, memories get reconsolidated each time they're brought up. If this is so and we can disrupt the process, then like magic, something else can potentially happen. Another well-known memory researcher named Joseph LeDoux said that:

"In short, once recalled, a memory is in a fragile state and susceptible to disruption. This has profound implications in PTSD research.

"If we could bring up traumatic memories associated with certain triggers, and then administer a drug that blocks protein synthesis, thus blocking Reconsolidation, we might improve the psychological outcome of thousands of returning veterans.

". . . the research so far suggests *it reduces the zing, takes the emotional valence out of the situation, rather than erases the memory itself.*"

How is this possible to do this without a drug? My colleague Richard Bruursema and I used the following display in our *Resetting the Fear Switch* 2015 published paper.

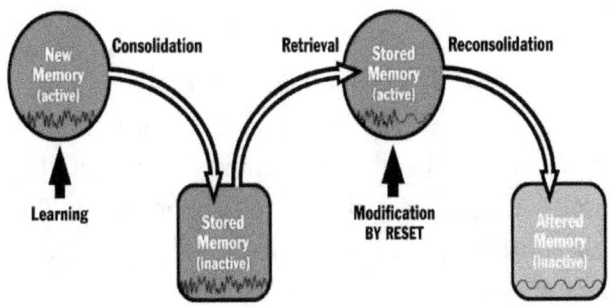

In the above illustration, a new memory is created through learning, even though the learning may come from a trauma of some kind. After it becomes firmly stored in the memory circuits of the brain, it is brought up again by intent or, in the case of PTSD, through triggers such as a particular scent, fireworks going off or a vehicle back firing.

Whenever this memory is retrieved it can be modified through neuromodulation means. Finally, note in the Altered Memory display that the electrical wave shape can be made different when it is subjected to 15 to 20 minutes of modulated sound.

Most remarkably and without exception, each of my patients undergoing this type of treatment gets to lose the emotional kick from the cobra when the interfering sound is provided while the 'limbic brain' is lit up. I personally imagine it as a switch being turned off, allowing the brain to RESET back to pre-trauma times. This is when the magic happens. The patient becomes her old self again.

Having observed this phenomenon numerous times, I have come to believe that it is possible to neutralize the emotional aspects of trauma. Through this procedure, my patients will not only experience relief of their symptoms, but will also become enabled to self-actualize.

They will have the opportunity to re-shape their self-perception that has been previously molded into a distorted form by their trauma. I have further come to believe that it will be much easier for my patients to transcend new fears when they are not linked to super-charged old emotional wounds.

When we can neutralize the trauma feelings, we also neutralize the 'poison within' thereby allowing the patient to begin the process of once again striving to attain his/her full potential and to become fully himself/herself. It is still amazing to me that executive functioning abilities seemingly return immediately permitting insight and perspective to emerge from within the patient.

A short case example might be helpful here to illustrate the treatment beginning with a rather straight-forward patient's response to an over-whelming fear that blocked her from under-going a necessary surgical procedure. Annie, a 36-year-old single female with 16+ years of education sought treatment due to a phobia related to her ongoing fear of needles and anesthesia.

Annie was unable to proceed with having blood drawn prior to a scheduled surgery for a rapidly developing ovarian cyst due to her being paralyzed with a devastating fear of needles and of being constrained. Annie's history revealed multiple major life traumas including rape and a near-death reaction following an injection of a medication that she was allergic to.

She was provided with a 15-minute intervention focused on perceptions that activated her fear of needles and immobilization. She reported that:

"I was so focused on the imagery that I didn't pay attention to the sound. I experienced a sense of layering and experienced them all at one time. There was no order or rhyme or reasoning but just fragments of experience.

"I felt like I was always above watching almost like a horror movie that I was engrossed in with all my senses. I had a memory of mom stung by bees - she almost died. It mirrors what I went through - like I inhaled her helplessness. It lived in me like a ghost. It depleted and was replaced by a sense of stability."

Annie was asked, following her treatment, to revisit part of it again. She reported the experience to be different with the sensation of being in a movie and now experiencing this story about a mother who was sad. She indicated that she was now ready to go through with the necessary operative procedure.

In her next visit, she reported that she had a surgical consult and felt a sense of confidence again. She perceived that her changes were dramatic. She scheduled and underwent her surgery recovering from this procedure within one day. Annie was so pleased with her results that she was ready to move on to other issues in her life. She is successfully regaining personal power and making continual progress in her personal life.

Recapping the earlier discussion, a specific type of modulated sound can connect (resonate) with a selectively activated (negatively charged) memory within the patient's Limbic System. The term resonate is quite complex.

Examples would include when a heavy truck goes by your home and your windows rattle. When this special sound is sustained for 15 to 20 minutes, the Reconsolidation process is interrupted and the brain resets to pre-trauma levels. This frees the patient from the accompanying emotional baggage produced by the traumatic event.

In many of my patients, remission occurs immediately. For some, it occurs gradually over 24 hours. Many patients develop insight and no longer appear to function in the immediacy of the previously feared event. This is when the amazing transformation occurs. This is when the intact person that you were prior to your trauma comes back into your life again.

Chapter Four:

Emerging Therapies

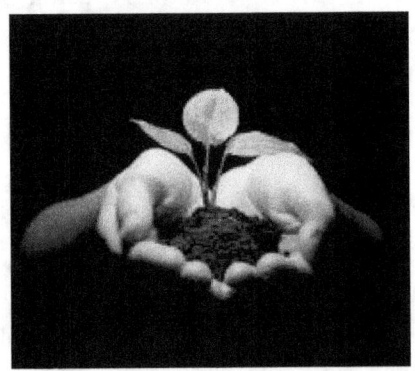

As discussed in GoodTherapy.org, Cognitive Behavioral Therapy (CBT) is a form of therapy in which the client and therapist form a trusted relationship in order to address issues causing the client distress. "Both therapist and client work together to discover the most pervasive issue and begin addressing that issue first.

"Cognitive behavioral therapy uses a practical approach in which the therapist helps the client understand the relationship between beliefs, feelings, and thoughts and the effect these have on behavior patterns and actions. The client learns that his or her perception will directly affect his or her reaction to certain conditions and circumstance and that this thought process is at the root of his or her behavior."

CBT encompasses many different approaches to create a flexible technique. "In CBT, clients are guided through their emotions using various tools. Therapists may employ techniques such as journaling, challenging beliefs, mindfulness or relaxation.

"Most people who receive this type of therapy usually do so for several months in sessions that last an hour at a time. The process of transformation is rarely fully recognized immediately. Clients learn how to replace negative thoughts and destructive behaviors with beneficial images, beliefs, and actions that will facilitate recovery.

"Clinicians use CBT for the treatment of mood issues in conjunction with mood-stabilizing medications. CBT is founded on the premise that our cognition, how we think of something, affects how we feel and how we act."

CBT addresses the cognitive, emotional, and behavioral aspects of a client with treatment provided through the following formats:

Exposure Therapy. This CBT therapy is designed to help people face and control their fear by exposing them to the trauma they experienced within a safe environment. The treatment utilizes mental imagery, writing, or might even include visits to the trauma site if possible.

Cognitive Restructuring. This therapy is designed to help people make sense of the traumatic experiences they have endured. An assumption made is that it is likely that the victim will remember the trauma event with feelings of guilt or shame even though the occurrence may not have been their fault. The therapeutic goal is to help the patient to look at the trauma in a realistic way.

Stress Inoculation Training. This therapy is focused on utilizing techniques such as meditation training, deep breathing procedures, etc., to reduce the symptoms of anxiety. Like cognitive restructuring, this treatment is designed to assist the patient to look at their traumatic experiences in a healthy way.

In his 2014 book, "The Body Keeps the Score: Brain, Mind, and Body in the Healing of Trauma," Dr. Bessel van der Kolk perceives of CBT as a form of Socratic dialogue that is designed to assist the patient to recognize maladaptive connections between their thoughts and their emotions.

He notes that, "Trauma has nothing whatsoever to do with cognition. It has to do with your body being reset to interpret the world as a dangerous place. That reset begins in the deep recesses of the brain with its most primitive structures, regions that no cognitive therapy can access. 'It's not something you can talk yourself out of." That view places him on the fringes of the psychiatric mainstream."

In regards to the above discussion, I am in complete and total agreement with Dr. van der Kolk and comfortably join him 'on the fringe'. However, I must go further because I have come to believe that both the body and the mind become stuck in a rigidified web of specific circuitry in the brain. I find it intriguing that he uses the word 'reset' in describing the body's reaction to trauma.

Let's start with a discussion in regards to Stress Inoculation Therapy. As reported by Harry Mills, Ph.D. et. al., Stress Inoculation Therapy (SIT) is intended to help patients prepare themselves to handle stressful events successfully and with a minimum of upset.

"The use of the term "inoculation" in SIT is based on the idea that a therapist is inoculating or preparing patients to become resistant to the effects of stressors in a manner similar to how a vaccination works to make patients resistant to the effects of particular diseases.

"Stress Inoculation Therapy is conceptually similar to relapse prevention methods used in addictions therapy. In SIT, patients are educated about stressful situations and the general nature of stress, the negative outcomes they may be vulnerable to experiencing when confronted with stress, and steps they can take to avoid those negative outcomes.

"At the conclusion of stress inoculation efforts, patients should feel like they can anticipate pitfalls that may occur during an event, and have a workable and practical plan in place for helping themselves avoid those pitfalls. In most instances, SIT consists of 8 to 15 sessions, plus booster and follow-up sessions, conducted over a 3-to-12-month period."

My perception (Lindenfeld) is that it is not realistic or practical to seek to prepare people for unexpected traumatic occurrences. The body instinctively reacts and for some, PTSD occurs. While one could justify training in handling stress in general, the cost and time factors preclude this as a primary intervention once trauma is locked into the neuronal system. Attempting to use this training as a front-line intervention for PTSD is analogous to closing the barn door after the horses have left the site and scattered.

In much the same way, another widely used procedure is called prolonged exposure therapy. I believe based on patient report and recent studies that, as it is currently applied, it will ultimately prove to be successful with PTSD in only one third of the unfortunate individuals who have to endure such a miserable treatment format.

An example of this torturous experience, which is claimed to be one of the 'gold standard' treatment interventions used by the Veterans Administration, is provided by David J. Morris. Because of copyright restrictions, I'm including the link for you to read the entire article. Selected excerpts are included.

http://opinionator.blogs.nytimes.com/2015/01/17/after-ptsd-more-trauma/#more-155563

"My first session began with my therapist, a graduate student finishing up his doctorate in clinical psychology. . . The promise of prolonged exposure is that your response to your trauma can be unlearned by telling the story of it over and over again.

". . . Over the course of our sessions, my therapist had me tell the story of the ambush dozens of times. .

. Given enough time and enough story 'reps,' when I opened my eyes again, I wouldn't feel forever perched on the precipice of a smoke-wreathed eternity. I wouldn't feel scared anymore.

"But after a month of therapy, I began to have problems. When I think back on that time, the word that comes to mind is 'nausea.' I felt sick inside, the blood hot in my veins. Never a good sleeper, I became an insomniac of the highest order. I couldn't read, let alone write.

". . . Following a heated discussion, in which I declared the therapy 'insane and dangerous' and my therapist ardently defended it, we decided to call it quits. . . Within a few weeks, my body returned to normal. My agitation subsided to the lower, simmering level it had been at before I went to the VA. I began once more to sleep, read and write. I never spoke about the I.E.D. attack again."

I find myself (Lindenfeld) horrified by the detailed account of a missed opportunity to have truly assisted this veteran to gain some semblance of remission from his PTSD condition. Had this psychology intern been aware of neuro-psychological consequences associated with trauma, he would have questioned his own ethics in proceeding with this patient in the manner he did based on the patient's frequently negative response to the intervention. And what of his supervisor?

Did his supervisor have any idea of the damage that was being done to this veteran? Perhaps the supervision was that of the 'hands off' variety where the intern gave his version of what was going on with this, 'highly resistant patient.'

How would the intern have addressed a now well-known and thoroughly researched shutdown of the Brocha's area of the brain (speech center) thereby limiting the veteran from fully articulating specifics of his varied encounters with trauma?

How would he account for a shutdown of executive functioning in the frontal lobe of the brain making it difficult for our veteran to 'connect the dots?' And how would he deal with the activated heart rate, elevated blood pressure and other physiological consequences of being frozen in a chronic fight, flight or freeze response? Ah well, I need to stop here as I feel the anger emerging within me.

Now let's contrast the above horror story with a RESET Therapy case example. I will introduce you to a friend that I will call Barry who is the firstborn of six children with his mother being initially a schoolteacher and then a government worker. His father was a U.S. Marshal and later a police officer.

He had PTSD from his World War II experience where he served as an Underwater Demolition Team member.

I have known Barry for many years now having worked with him as a colleague and continuing my relationship with him as a friend. When approached about using RESET Therapy, he thoughtfully stated that nothing else had been able to alter his frequent struggle with PTSD, "so why not give it a try." Barry was willing to provide a history of his developmental difficulties as well as discussing the insults and humiliations he experienced within the context of his schooling and military experience.

"My dad saw a great deal of action and had a lot of bad experiences during that particular war. At home, he was overwhelmed with children as they had six of them. I was the firstborn and was early diagnosed as having nervous child syndrome which was later changed to pervasive developmental disorder.

"At five years of age, I was diagnosed with Tourette's syndrome. I had other health complications including scarlet fever later followed by rheumatic fever that was followed by Sydenham's chorea which produced uncoordinated jerking movements primarily affecting my face, hands and feet. A year after that, I developed Tourette's syndrome.

"In the middle of all this, I was sexually abused by a female cousin who was three years older than me. My father didn't know how to deal with me and my mother was bipolar so neither of them really knew how to cope with a child with my complicated condition. They would hit me a lot to keep me from ticking which made it worse. I carried the secret of the sexual abuse because my cousin was close to my parents.

"Basically, I got bullied all the way through my school years including college. When I was, younger I was small but then had a growth spurt and was big. Seem like I got into a lot of fights and got into a lot of trouble because people would tease me because of my tics and because I didn't know how to interact socially.

"It wasn't until I was 27 that I was ultimately diagnosed with an Asperger's condition. When I graduated from high school, I went into the military going through boot camp with my Tourette's condition. After completing boot camp, I went out on leave and was attacked by drug dealers. My army friends, who unknown to me were prior drug dealers brought me to a house they frequented previously.

"The guys there were active drug dealers and were mad that the guys brought me there. The people ran me down and gave me a shot of barbiturates in my side which knocked me out. They brought me to the airport and put me on a plane back to Great Lakes.

"When I got back, I told them the whole story but they didn't believe me so they searched my locker and found what they called contraband in my locker. To this day, I don't what it was. They arrested me and put me in the brig. The military police took my sea bag and dumped it on the floor and said, "Guys, here is a loser. I got attacked by three other people in the brig and they raped me.

"I finally got away from them and grabbed a piece of metal off the bunk bed and beat all of them half to death. One guy, I broke his skull wide open. I went to the bathroom and washed the blood off my hands. I put the metal from the bunk bed back up and lay down and then the Marine Military Police came back in.

"Here were these guys laying all over the floor and one guy up against the wall with his skull busted open. They took him to the hospital and the other two guys said they fell. Nobody would tell on me but I was absolutely traumatized by all of this. I was so very naïve, not being able to interact with people and this whole thing just flooded me.

"For years, it's been on my mind but I had it pushed back. After Katrina, it flooded me again. I was having nightmares, daytime intrusions, and terrible panic and anxiety as well as physical pain. I was treated for seven years for PTSD at the VA with no measurable change and then, after the advice of my friend, I used RESET Therapy. After one treatment, the majority of my symptoms were gone and I continued to use it prophylactically and now there are no remaining symptoms of PTSD left to haunt me.

"With my schooling, I completed all but my dissertation in biological and physiological psychology. I proceeded to spend four years at Georgetown studying psychophysiology relationships. When I first heard about RESET Therapy, I was very skeptical. Amazingly, after I tried it, I had immediate relief of my PTSD symptoms.

"I completed the protocol and had complete and total relief from the past traumas in my life with a total of five sessions. I know that this intervention has to be tapping into the Hippocampus and the Amygdala but I haven't the slightest clue as to what causes the healing aspect of it. I do think it has a reconsolidation effect."

As Barry noted, he had extensive training in biological and physiological psychology. He was quite skeptical about the treatment yet he reported total remission of his Complex PTSD condition in five applications of RESET.

Let's discuss what's causing the healing aspect of it. Remember the neuronal model of activation when PTSD is flaring as captured in an fMRI and earlier described in Chapter Four?

When RESET Therapy is involved we would expect the following consequences: a greater connection to frontal lobe executive functioning ability resulting in increasing levels of insight; increase in the patient's ability to articulate due to the Brocha's area coming back online; a diminishment of the fight, flight or freeze mode of functioning should begin to be evidenced; a reduction in delusional material and or flashbacks should be reported. Clearly, diminishment of the fight, flight or freeze response occurred for Barry.

At this point in time, the discussion regarding treatment for PTSD, Eye Movement Desensitization and Reprocessing Therapy (EMDR) appears to be the closest to RESET Therapy in its effects on the circuitry of the brain. This treatment was originated by psychologist, Dr. Francine Shapiro in 1987.

While experiencing an incidental disturbing thought, she became aware that rapid lateral eye movement reduced the intensity of her focus. Consequently, a scientific study with trauma victims was conducted in 1988 with the research published in the *Journal of Traumatic Stress* in 1989.

"Shapiro noted that, when she was experiencing a disturbing thought, her eyes were involuntarily moving rapidly. She noticed further that, when she brought her eye movements under voluntary control while thinking a traumatic thought, anxiety was reduced."

"Shapiro developed EMDR therapy for posttraumatic stress disorder. She speculated that traumatic events "upset the excitatory/inhibitory balance in the brain, causing a pathological change in the neural elements.

"EMDR therapy uses a structured eight-phase approach to address the past, present, and future aspects of a traumatic or distressing memory. The therapy process and procedures are guided by the Adaptive Information Processing Model which proposed that EMDR facilitates the processing of traumatic material enabling an adaptive resolution.

"During the therapy, the most commonly used intervention is to have the patient focus on unsettling material while visually tracking the therapist's finger rapidly moving back and forth. The originator of this therapy postulated that it enables access to trauma memories leading to more adaptive processing, reduction in emotional disturbance and the emergence of insight."

Sounds like the neuronal model, doesn't it? Seemingly, the treatment opens access to loosely associated memories and images from the past. When successful, the patient experiences their prior trauma as past rather than present.

Where EMDR is similar to RESET Therapy is that talking is discouraged during the treatment process with focus directed towards inner emerging material. Both therapies do not necessarily require a trusting, therapeutic relationship.

Where they differ is that in RESET Therapy, the patient is asked to experience the targeted trauma fully and totally while listening to the neuromodulation sound. With EMDR, the patient focuses on a trauma fragment that emerges consequent to experiencing rapid eye movement.

My personal experience with both approaches is that RESET Therapy proceeds much quicker with less preparatory time required. While there are numerous other body focused therapies currently available, these will not be discussed in detail in this book. Rather, the reader is referred to Dr. Bessel A. van der Kolk 2014 book entitled: "The Body Keeps the Score: Brain, Mind, and Body in the Healing of

Trauma" for a more detailed account of these interventions.

Chapter Five:

Fight, Flight or Freeze

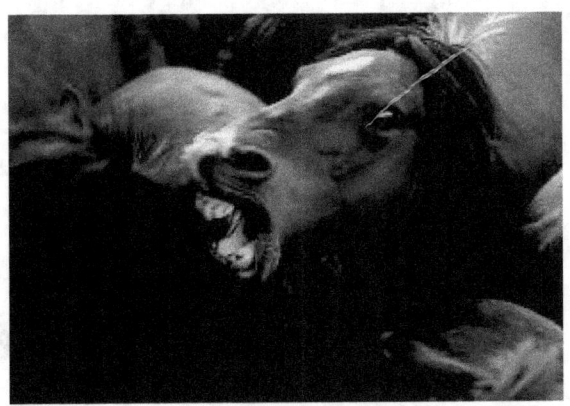

Some of you may find this chapter to be somewhat too technical, so I've decided to include a case study provided by a Vietnam veteran we'll refer to as Joe. A year after being evaluated for a VA disability rating, Joe decided to seek treatment with me stating that,

****

I've come to see you because I've been having bad dreams this past year and my wife has become afraid to touch me. If a car backfires, it kicks off panic reactions in me.

night In 1966 while we were spending our first in Vietnam at Camp Bravo, a rocket came in and blew up an aviation fuel tank. It lit up the whole world. They gave us a mattress to lay down underneath so no one could see us, as if that damn mattress would change anything.

the One time the Viet Cong (VC) attacked while we were crossing a bridge. The VC blew up bridge behind us. A lieutenant and the others were up front in a Jeep. The lieutenant got rolled in a ditch, and got killed with a concussion grenade. He had one little drop of blood on his nose, that's all, but the rest of his insides was gel. I just can't get that drop of blood out of my mind.

A year later, with many combat missions under his belt, Joe returned to California with his unit.

me That's when the hell really hit the fire. When we arrived, there were demonstrators. We got called every name in the book. They called baby killer, they spat on me and they threw rocks at me. These damn people sent me there to do a job, and then they treated me and my brothers like trash.

When he returned to his unit after a personal leave, Joe was assigned burial detail for soldiers who had died in Vietnam.

> We'd be standing in formation around a casket in his hometown for this guy that fell and died in Vietnam. But, yet the American people treated us like shit.

****

With some animals, when predators attack, they will immediately freeze or 'play dead.' The response includes a restriction of activity when the animal perceives that there is little chance of escaping. Little focus has been directed scientifically in regard to this tendency in humans.

The survival response starts in the emotional center of the brain referred to as the Limbic System. The Amygdala, which plays a primary role in the processing of memory, decision-making and emotional reactivity becomes activated releasing neuronal messaging to the Hypothalamus whose primary function is to maintain the body's status quo system-wide. This organ produces many of the body's essential hormones which govern functions such as temperature regulation, thirst, hunger, sleep, mood, sex drive, and the release of other hormones within the body.

This area of the brain houses the pituitary gland and other glands in the body. During stress, chemical messengers trigger the production of cortisol which prepares muscles throughout the body for rapid response. This also increases blood pressure, blood sugar, and suppresses the immune system in order to attain a boost of energy to meet the real or imagined 'attack.'

****

and

on

Joe said he was bothered that a close friend former neighbor who served in World War II committed suicide. "He took a 22 rifle, set it his car, and pulled the trigger." When I asked if Joe has considered hurting himself, he said he has, but stopped short of forming a plan. "I know I would have, it would have happened. I was very nervous, and had a bad attitude. If it weren't for RESET Therapy, I wouldn't be here."

****

The release of adrenaline or noradrenaline triggers many rapid physical reactions related to preparing the organism for extreme muscular responses. They may include a number of the following responses: bladder relaxation, dilation of blood vessels to muscles, diminished hearing, erection inhibition, flushing or paling, increased heart rate and breathing action, inhibited tear production and salivation, metabolic energy increase, peripheral vision loss, pupil dilation, selective blood vessel constriction, shaking, slowing of the digestive process, sphincter effect, and spinal reflex disinhibition.

****

In his first RESET Therapy session, Joe reported that:

It all went away – It faded out. What happened is there but it didn't affect me that much. When we first started, my heart was going 90 miles a minute. My muscles were tense and tears started rolling. Then it wasn't there anymore. The emotions didn't come with it! I'm feeling at peace now."

Joe was skeptical that his results would be only temporary, so he asked if it would be alright to return for a number of follow-up sessions. He returned a week later reporting that he was sleeping better.

Previously, I was waking up every hour. I used to wake sitting straight up. I'm also remembering more things now that I previously couldn't think about."

****

Males tend to respond to a critical situation with aggression first (fight). Females are inclined to seek an escape route (flight), try to defuse the situation, or engage in nurturing efforts such as displaying protective behavior towards their children. These responses persist in present times, however; broader outlets have emerged in modern men and women such as substance abuse as a means of avoiding conflict (flight).

With PTSD, the fight, flight or freeze response doesn't stop after the initiating event as the sufferer is constantly triggered by threatening internal or external stimuli such as nightmares or a car backfiring. This is caused by the hyperarousal of the Autonomic Nervous System that becomes the driver behind varied symptoms referred to as flashbacks, dissociative tendencies and the freeze response. The listed varied symptoms provided above produce complex thinking difficulties (part of the brain that controls decisions & taking rational action), sleep difficulties, sexual dysfunction, appetite disturbance, etc.

****

Joe's wife accompanied him to his second treatment reporting that:

> He's been really mean to me and moody for such a long time." During his 20 minutes of RESET Therapy, Joe targeted all the newly emerging memories that had surfaced into his awareness. He reported that: "I went through it all and can't think of anything else. I'm feeling relaxed and could fall asleep right now."

The following session, Joe reported that he had been feeling good all week.

> Vietnam stuff didn't even enter my mind! It used to happen 3 to 4 times a day. Something would trigger it – now it's not there. A lawnmower backfired and I didn't even jump – that's very unusual for me. I'm getting more energy now. My emotions have settled down and I don't feel like I have to cry anymore."

****

As noted earlier, the arousal function appears to be closely arbitrated by the Limbic System, which is primarily engaged in survival efforts including the fight, flight or freeze response as well as the processing of memory. It is also closely engaged with the Autonomic Nervous System that controls vital organs in the body such as the heart, lungs, bowel and pupils.

The Sympathetic Nervous System, when aroused by hormones released by the Limbic System, triggers the body for the instinctive attack, avoidance or immobilization reaction. These survival reactions are instinctive and situation-dependent. If neither running away nor counter-attacking is possible, a reflexive form of reality-alteration occurs that produces a slowing of time in the victim's mind, resulting in a dissociative sense of diminished fear and pain. If this should become chronic, in essence, the fear circuit has become stuck in the 'ON' position.

****

Joe's wife reported:

> He's doing better and not jumping up and
> down every time I ask him to do something. He sleeps better – no moaning. He doesn't sit

straight up in bed suddenly at night. He has more patience with me now when we shop." Joe added that, "We've been married for 52 years, and she's been through it all. I would give the world to her if I could."

****

The Limbic System's Amygdala region contains emotionally-charged memories, while the Hippocampus appears to be involved in the storage of place and time-related events. When the Hippocampus is stuck in the **"ON"** position, its function becomes inactive, de-linking it from the past, and seemingly causing the sufferer to relive incidents over and over again in the present.

Another phenomenon that may occur is a shattering of awareness called dissociation. This may begin with forgetting that attains a level of amnesia extending to a complete fragmentation of the personality that is now called Dissociative Identity Disorder formerly known as Multiple Personality Disorder. In summary, the freeze victim of PTSD experiences an overall numbing of sensation, distorted sense of time and absence of fear, replacing it with a seemingly altered state of consciousness that dramatically alters her/his quality of life's experiences.

Another case example of a form of freeze response is presented in changes experienced by one of Asheville, North Carolina's veterans, Ron LaPointe, following treatment with RESET Therapy (Reconsolidation Enhancement by Stimulation of Emotional Triggers).

Ron had also served honorably in Vietnam's Central Highlands in 1967 and found himself when arriving back in Los Angeles, being greeted by protesters who were screaming obscenities and waving hateful signs at him and his military brothers. He consequently flew to New York to visit his sister intending to take a train to Long Island from Grand Central Station. While walking, a bus backfired.

****

I dropped to my knees hitting the pavement as my arms came up to cover my head. That's when I realized that I had a problem. It's taken me 44 years to be able to talk about this.

After returning to his family's farm in Maine, he proceeded to burn his uniform in a trash can because he felt ashamed of his service.

I didn't want to share my experience with my family or other veterans because I didn't want to go on reliving what happened to me in Vietnam. Regarding the treatment, I was skeptical at first but the problem is gone. I can now walk the streets and if a plane or helicopter is overhead, I don't have to dive into the street anymore! Helicopters, gunshots, etc. no longer trigger a protective response that I have tolerated for decades.

****

You will be learning more about this intriguing treatment known as RESET Therapy in the next chapter where the details of the intervention will be provided. Furthermore, you will be provided with case examples throughout this book in order to give you the opportunity to appreciate how empowering it is to experience a total transformation of your mind, body and spirit.

Chapter Six:

No More Flashbacks or Nightmares

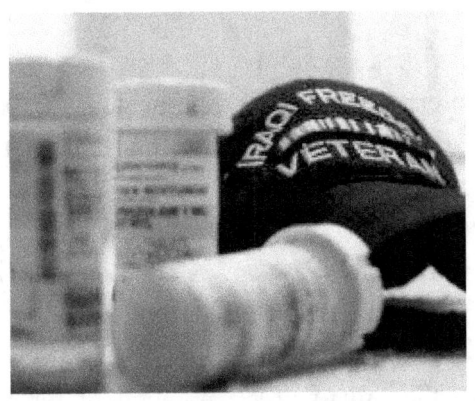

In 1980, the American Psychiatric Association (APA) added PTSD to the third edition of its Diagnostic and Statistical Manual of Mental Disorders (DSM-III) classification scheme. In its initial formulation, a traumatic event was conceptualized as a catastrophic stressor that was outside the range of usual human experience.

The framers of the original PTSD diagnosis had in mind events such as war, torture, rape, the Nazi Holocaust, the atomic bombings of Hiroshima and Nagasaki, natural disasters (such as earthquakes, hurricanes, and volcano eruptions) and human-made disasters (such as factory explosions, airplane crashes, and automobile accidents). They considered traumatic events to be clearly different from the very painful stressors that constitute the normal vicissitudes of life such as divorce, failure, rejection, serious illness, financial reverses, and the like.

Dr. Peter Levine, a contemporary expert in regards to trauma is referenced in his comprehensive 2010 book titled: *"An Unspoken Voice – How the Body Releases Trauma and Restores Goodness"* points out that, "current (DSM-III) terminology, (was) derived largely from the Vietnam war, as posttraumatic stress disorder.

"As PTSD, the universal phenomena of terror and paralysis - in which the nervous system has been strained to the breaking point, leaving body, psyche and soul shattered - is now fully sanitized as a medical 'disorder.' With its own convenient acronym, and serving the dispassionate nature of science, the archetypal response to carnage has now been artificially severed from its ravaging origins.

"Where it was once aptly conveyed by the terms *fright paralysis* and *shell shock*, it is now simply a disorder, an objectified collection of concrete and measurable symptoms; a diagnosis amenable to vested research protocols, detached insurance companies and behavioral treatment strategies.

"While this nomenclature provides objective scientific legitimacy to the soldier's very real suffering, it also safely separates doctor from patient. The 'healthy' ('protected') doctor treats the 'ill' patient. This approach disempowers and marginalizes the sufferer, adding to his or her sense of alienation and despair. Less noticed is the likely burnout in the unprotected healer, who has been artificially hoisted on to a precarious pedestal as false prophet.

". . . Nonetheless, the medical model persists. It (arguably) functions fairly effectively with diseases like diabetes and cancer, where the doctor holds all of the knowledge and dictates the necessary interventions for a sick patient. This is not, however, a useful paradigm for trauma healing. Rather than being a disease in the classical sense, trauma is instead a profound *experience* of 'dis-ease' or 'dis-order.' What is called for here is a cooperative and restorative process with the doctor as an assisting guide and midwife.

"A doctor who insists on retaining his or her protected role as 'healthy healer' remain separate, defending himself or herself against the ultimate helplessness that lurks, phantom like, in all of our lives. Cut off from his or her own feelings, such a doctor will not be able to join with the sufferer.

"Missing will be the crucial collaboration in containing, processing and integrating the patient's horrible sensations, images and emotions. The sufferer will remain starkly alone, holding the very horrors that have overwhelmed him and broken down his capacity to self-regulate and grow."

I am in full agreement with Dr. Levine's premise in the above paragraphs. I wonder at times if my professional colleagues shy away from engaging trauma patients in treatment due to their own instinctive fear of not being able to handle the emotional charge that this type of patient brings into the therapy room.

Alternatively, when faced with the potential tidal wave of emotions that this patient brings to the fore, how does one reconcile it with the restrictions imposed by the managed care system with its inherent limitations? An example of this was noted in Chapter One with therapist Katherine Therrell's reference to, "his Employee Assistance Program authorized 6 pre-approved counseling sessions to try to resolve this problem."

Thus, I believe that a number of factors result in self-imposed limitations preventing therapists from fully engaging in treatment with trauma patients. Furthermore, and here is where I disagree with Dr. Levine, the empathic qualifications that he clearly possesses and advises as being necessary to take on this type of client, may be beyond the reach of many practicing therapists.

Furthermore, although these qualities are clearly important, in RESET Therapy when done properly, the neuro-modulatory sound resonates with the patient's trauma, the therapist doesn't necessarily have to. My concern about this is the inherent danger of the therapist's repeated exposure to trauma material that leads to the development of secondary PTSD. Dr. Levine notes that:

"Biological, or postural tuning is also the foundation for the 'therapeutic resonance' that is vitally important in helping people heal from trauma. A therapist who is not aware of how his or her own body reacts to (i.e., resonates with) the fear, rage, helplessness and shame in another person will not be able to guide clients by *tracking* their sensations and navigating them safely through the sometimes treacherous (albeit therapeutic) waters of traumatic sensations.

"At the same time, by learning how to attract the wrong sensations, therapists can avoid *absorbing* the fear, rage and helplessness of their clients. It is important to understand that when therapists perceive that they must protect themselves from their client's sensations and emotions, they consciously block those clients from therapeutically experiencing them.

By distancing ourselves from their anguish, we distance ourselves from them and from the fears they are struggling with.

"To take a self-protective stance is to abandon our clients precipitately. At the same time, we also greatly increase the likelihood of their exposure to secondary or vicarious traumatization and burnout. Therapists must learn, from their own successful encounters with their own traumas, to stay present with their clients. This is the reason healing trauma must necessarily engage the awareness of the living, sensing, 'knowing' body in *both* client and therapist." ("In an Unspoken Voice,")

In contrast, I believe that too much closeness or "therapeutic resonance" produces burnout in therapists. As I referenced in Chris Morkides' article in Chapter Four, (May 2009 in *Counseling Today)* "Mental health counseling is a demanding profession. Listening to the same sorts of problems all day long may result in counselor fatigue, which is usually characterized by feelings of detachment, dehumanization and exhaustion in dealing with clients.

"A related risk is compassion fatigue, in which the efforts of helping a client traumatize the counselor. I also noted that: There is a way to fix this secondary PTSD problem. The primary way is by allowing the therapist to experience and take part in facilitating quick and sometimes immediate restoration of normal functioning in the patient.

Secondly, he/she must be spared from the highly charged expressive narrative that is emotionally conveyed by the patient rather directly from the limbic brain. When the above components occur, the therapist's empathic skill set can be fully utilized to assist the patient with his or her transformative therapeutic process.

A case example is presented here to clarify my perspective. Trudie B. experienced military sexual trauma (MST) in 2003 within the context of her military service. When she reported sexual abuse to her chain of command, disciplinary action was taken against her rather than the perpetrator. To complicate matters further, Trudie was also involved in a IED explosion that took place on Christmas day 2005 which caused additional emotional damage to her.

This Veteran endorsed having difficulties with authoritarian males beginning in her childhood. Over the course of time, following her sexual abuse and I.E.D. experience, she experienced two failed marriages and with two young children was struggling with her third. Lack of intimacy had become a central issue within this context.

Given the above circumstances Trudie experienced much relief in not having to verbalize the rape circumstances before an authoritative male figure. This enabled her to fully engage in the internalized focus of activating all of her senses related to that trauma. I refer to this as 'lighting up the target.'

The treatment process I refer to as RESET Therapy will be described in detail later in this book. My point here is that due to the effects of her treatment, Trudie was able to quickly release the emotional and physical consequences of her experiences. This enabled her to 'reset' her trauma circuitry backed to a balanced state in a way that occurs when one reboots a computer.

From the therapist's perspective, this treatment format allowed me to be a supportive figure enabling a healing, transformation to occur within the patient without disrupting the process itself. I become the guide that Dr. Levine envisioned as well as the initiating agent of bodily release of trauma that Dr. van der Kolk refers to.

At the same time, it wasn't necessary for me to become engrossed in the details of her trauma experiences nor to interpret what meanings she derived. I was able to later provide her with expectation related to her release. For example, I informed her that her body might 'shake, rattle and roll' as the muscles were finally set free from the protective stance they had assumed.

We visit Dr. Bessel A. van der Kolk, who was featured in the New York Times Magazine, *The Health Issue*, in an article written by Jeneen Interlandi on May 22, 2014 entitled, "A Revolutionary Approach to Treating PTSD". Selective aspects of this article are included in this text because they fully complement the underlying neuroscientific principles that form the basis for RESET as a comprehensive treatment.

While honoring the extensive work that Dr. van der Kolk has accomplished, I (Lindenfeld) perceive that his perspective has not gone far enough. This will be clarified further in later discussion.

We begin with the reporter's comment that: "Dr. van der Kolk has come to believe that the way to treat psychological trauma is not through the mind but through the body. 'In so many cases, it was patients' bodies that had been grossly violated, and it was their bodies that had failed them — legs had not run quickly enough, arms had not pushed powerfully enough, voices had not screamed loudly enough to evade disaster. And it was their bodies that now crumpled under the slightest of stresses — that dove for cover with every car alarm or saw every stranger as an assailant in waiting.

"How could their minds possibly be healed if they found the bodies that encased those minds so intolerable? The single most important issue for traumatized people is to find a sense of safety in their own bodies,' van der Kolk says.

"Trauma victims, van der Kolk likes to say, are alienated from their bodies by a cascade of events that begins deep in the brain with an almond-shaped structure known as the amygdala. When faced with a threat, the amygdala triggers a fight-or-flight response, which includes the release of a flood of hormones. This response usually persists until the threat is vanquished. But if the threat isn't vanquished — if we can't fight or flee — the amygdala, which can be thought of as the body's smoke detector, keeps sounding the alarm.

"We keep producing stress hormones, which in turn wreak havoc on the rest of our bodies. It's similar to what happens in chronic stress, except that in traumatic stress, the memories of the traumatic event invade patients' subconscious thoughts, sending them back into fight-or-flight mode at the slightest provocation. Therapists and patients refer to this as being 'reactivated.'

"In the short term, patients avoid the pain it causes by 'dissociating.' That is, they take leave of their bodies, so much so that they often cannot describe their own physical sensations. This happens a lot in therapy, van der Kolk says. . .

"In the long term, they become experts in self-numbing. They use food, exercise, work — or worse, drugs and alcohol — to stifle physical discomfort. The longer they do this, the more difficult it becomes to remain present in any given moment. The goal of treatment should be to resolve this disconnect. If we can help our patients tolerate their own bodily sensations, they'll be able to process the trauma themselves', he says."

In his 2014 book, "The Body Keeps the Score: Brain, Mind, and Body in the Healing of Trauma.", Dr. van der Kolk notes that: "In order to regain control over yourself, you need to revisit the trauma: Sooner or later you need to confront what is happening to you, but only after you feel safe and will not be re-traumatized by it.

The first order of business is to find ways to cope with feeling overwhelmed by the sensations and emotions associated with the past. . . The fundamental issue in resolving traumatic stress is to restore the proper balance between the rational and emotional brains, so that you can feel in charge of how you respond and how you conduct your life. . .

If you want to change posttraumatic reactions, we have to access the emotional brain and do 'Limbic system therapy': repairing faulty alarm systems and restoring the emotional brain to its ordinary job of being a quiet background presence that takes care of the housekeeping of the body, ensuring that you eat, sleep, connect with intimate partners, protect your children, and defend against danger.

. . Traumatized people are often afraid of feeling. It is not so much the perpetuators (who, hopefully, are no longer around to hurt them) but their own physical sensations that now are the enemy.

"Apprehension about being hijacked by uncomfortable sensations keep the brain frozen and the mind shut. Even though the trauma is a thing of the past, the emotional brain keeps generating sensations that make the sufferer feel scared and helpless. It's not surprising that so many trauma survivors are compulsive eaters and drinkers, fear making love, and avoid many social activities: Their sensory world is largely off limits."

As you would expect, I have the same perspective with this set of beliefs. While it is certainly humane to wish to, "restore the proper balance between the rational and emotional brains" the real-life question is, what does it takes in time, resources and professional skill to accomplish this objective?

If it were possible to achieve this quickly through sound that resonates with the patient's trauma thereby blocking the restoration of the emotional aspects of trauma, shouldn't we explore this break-through intervention with all the current sophisticated brain imaging tools currently available to us such as the fMRI?

Both Drs. Levine and van der Kolk perceive that the methodology necessary to treat PTSD is through the body in order to quiet and calm the limbic brain. Based on this belief, they are inclined to address the body first through varied interventions that approach it in non-verbal ways. Alternatively, I have come to the conclusion that 'resetting the fear switch' in the brain creates a transformative alteration in both the body and the mind restoring completeness rapidly and fully.

Let's look at another yet another example of RESET therapy with a veteran who was stuck in the chronic anger/fight stage of his PTSD condition. Robert served honorably in the Vietnam War as a gunner who was thrust headfirst into horrific experiences that are difficult for a human being to imagine. He has suffered for nearly 50 years from the after effects of this experience, unable to shake the traumatic memories that have haunted him.

He has struggled to cope with a sleep disorder, drug use and overwhelming anxiety further complicated by misdiagnosis, unsuccessful therapy, multiple hospitalizations, and numerous medications that left him numb and devoid of his personality. He is like tens of thousands of other vets who suffer in silence.

In Robert's Diagnostic Intake he revealed that, "Things would flare-up and I would get into fights. I did drugs. I stopped taking my medications because I was still having flashbacks." His wife reported that her husband was quite mean toward her and that she was at her wit's end trying to deal with his endless anger and rage.

Robert joined the Marines in exchange for having criminal charges against him dropped in court. From Camp Pendleton, he was deployed to Vietnam and a couple of weeks later he was called into combat as a mortar gunman. In one gruesome instance, Robert described how he was directed to help about 20 wounded Marines in the field aboard a chopper and then he had to collect the bodies of those that died whose remains lay in the field.

> We packed all the bodies in a pile as we were fighting and a round came in and hit them. There were body parts everywhere. We had to gather them up. I've had lots of flashbacks of picking up the pieces.

Another incident involved firing rounds of white phosphorous on houses after they had tried to evacuate inhabitants.

> There were many people that just wouldn't come out. When we hit the houses all the kids and others started coming out. Some were killed and some died later. Word was that all of them died. That has haunted me for years and years.

> After I got back from Vietnam I had flashbacks and nightmares. For 15 to 20 years I was nothing but an alcoholic and a drug addict. I would bolt upright from sleep at night terrified because I thought I was in combat.

His flashbacks started a few months after returning. Some of the triggers were the smells of gunpowder, burning flesh or decomposition and fireworks.

Robert was hospitalized over 30 times after being diagnosed by the VA as being paranoid schizophrenic and a psychopath. I carefully reviewed DSM-IV criteria for PTSD within the context of the patient's symptomatology in contrast with criteria necessary for a diagnosis of paranoid schizophrenia. It became glaringly apparent that this patient had been misdiagnosed and provided with medications that did not address the symptoms of his primary diagnosis of PTSD.

Given his diagnosis and negative prior experience from traditional psychotherapy and medication I chose to utilize RESET-Anxiety as an initial treatment of choice. After carefully tuning the device's sound to resonate with one of his trauma targets, Robert was provided with a 15-minute intervention utilizing this neuromodulation treatment 'while lighting up the target'.

On his return visit one week later, Robert reported that,

> I was thinking about the event and all but it seemed more peaceful. I haven't had any nightmares or flashbacks compared to previously having them 2 to 3 times per week.

His wife reported that her husband had done some work on the car rather than just sitting despondently in the house.

> Now he talks again and is carrying on conversations. He didn't do that before. He would just lay in bed with a dark look on his face eating and watching TV all the time. His communication is getting better and he is

getting back to the way he used to be. He helps with the chores. The very first treatment he had was like a miracle. He went home, slept well, didn't jerk awake, didn't jump up awake slamming, screaming, looking like someone was going to kill him.

Robert perceived that he was doing better with his Vietnam issues and consequently, he was encouraged to test his limits by watching war movies focusing on this era. He was seen in follow-up one week later and reported that:

> I watched a war story and it didn't bother me at all. When I wake up I feel great! I don't argue over any little things anymore. I was talking with a guy about Vietnam and it didn't bother me.

His wife noted that, "He hasn't been having any nightmares and doesn't jerk anymore at night. Overall he is improving but I'm concerned about his gambling problem."

Robert selected his next target, which, at his wife's insistence, was focused on his urge to gamble. On his return the following week he reported that, "I don't want to play anymore. The charge in it for me is gone."

His wife added that, "His whole attitude is changed. He seems to be doing marvelously well." A final therapy target was selected which consisted of his resentment at his father for favoring his older sister and brother.

"My father met me at the airport when I came back from Vietnam. That was the first time he actually ever seemed to be glad to see me. I was close to my mom but she died when I was 15. I probably never got over her death."

In his final appointment, he relayed that he was feeling better about this matter and was now able to go with things on his own. He has been followed since therapy through telephone contact and his PTSD has remained in remission for well over one year at the time of the writing of this article.

The above case illustrates the complexity frequently seen in Vietnam era patients with chronic PTSD and other accompanying mental health issues. Robert's rapid response to this unique therapy is quite typical for the preponderance of my veterans and civilians who have undergone this treatment for trauma.

Amazingly, the majority of my patients undergoing this intervention remain in remission from their PTSD symptomatology. A cautionary note is required here in regards to Complex PTSD which requires ongoing intervention. The treatment process in this type of case is expedited through the use of RESET Therapy but does not typically resolve as rapidly as does target specific cases.

Clearly, therapeutic skill is a necessary ingredient for those professionals offering RESET Therapy to our warriors that wish to return to a peace-time environment following their service in dangerous settings. This is not a do-it-yourself project.

A competent therapist guide, skilled and knowledge-able about treatment procedures, is essential to turn of the 'fear switch' permanently and completely. With this in mind, my mission is incomplete until enough licensed healers are thoroughly trained, certified and readily available throughout the nation to meet your needs.

In the interim, I will build the structure that meets the criteria of scientific validity to attain this objective. This is my commitment to you and to your loved ones as we push ahead with making this knowledge available.

Chapter Seven:

Semper Fidelis

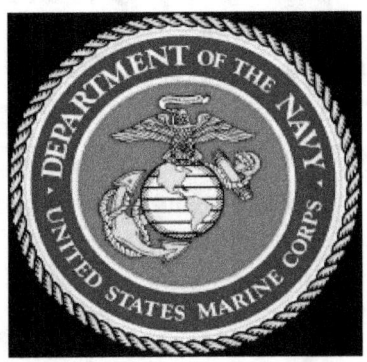

This case study differs from the ones you've read previously as it falls under the heading of Complex PTSD. Yes, it is about a wounded veteran who came back with PTSD. However, in Paul's case, his wounds added additional layers to those he incurred through childhood and a troublesome adolescence.

Paul was raised within a badly damaged family. Therapists speak of a 'weak core personality' or difficulty during the 'attachment phase' in the development of the personality in cases such as this. While RESET Therapy is still remarkably successful with PTSD, in complex cases it must be provided in an ongoing series of sessions with a greater level of support than required in non-complex cases.

My treatment relationship with Paul was further complicated because we lived in different locations. Because of this, we primarily used long-distance communication conducted through email and phone. We were able to do this successfully since he had a BAUD as well as local therapeutic support. You will hear not only Paul's story, but also that of his wife, Alice, whose revelations give us a deeper perspective on what it's like to live with someone with PTSD.

'Paul's Story'

"I had a difficult and traumatic childhood including bad memories of living in Pittsburgh in a small three story house with my step-sister and two younger brothers. My mother was separated from my father most of the time that we lived there which for me was from about age four to eleven.

"Most of these days seemed very intense and stressful. Mother was not able to cope with four children, no husband and little financial support. She was born in Russia in 1917 and my understanding is that she had near death experiences during the Bolshevik regime.

"Mom told me that when she was two or three years old, the Bolshevik's were rounding up Jewish people to kill them. She and her family escaped while hiding in a barn. Eventually the eldest brother helped the family escape to Cuba and then to immigrate to the USA.

"Mom was terrified of her oldest brother and told stories about how she literally peed in her pants when he would exhibit anger toward her. Mom was in a frequent state of fight or flight, panic and worry, and acted out toward me with anger, rage and cursing.

"She admitted to me and my brothers when we were older that she hated us three boys because to her, we represented our father. She said that she resented him for coercing her to have children and then leaving her alone to raise us.

"Mom always cried out for her older brother or sister or even people in the neighborhood to help her. When she would break down and cry she would say, "I can't take it anymore, I can't handle this." As an adult I came to believe the same.

"When I got stressed I learned to give up in frustration and believed that I might die because I could not take it anymore – just like my mom. As a result, I had a lot of anxiety.

"As I got older, about seven to ten, I was made to be responsible for my two younger brothers. I frequently got blamed for everything that went wrong being blamed for what they did or didn't do. My cleaning was never good enough and I was never good enough! Mom constantly used me to release all her anger and hate.

"I was frequently cursed at, hit at, berated, and screamed at for many years. I remember being terrified when she tied me to the boiler in the basement. It was dark and I was very afraid that I would die alone and no one would help me.

"This started my worst fear that has been with me all my life: that of being frightened to death to be alone. I thought that in that basement I would die and no one would help me. I eventually imagined I was dead and that way she couldn't hurt me anymore.

"I never expressed how I felt but usually kept my mouth shut and mostly imagined I was talking to mom in my head or someone else. I was always trying to please mother to gain her acceptance and love, but it never seemed like I was good enough or I did enough.

"I learned how to shut down my emotions and voice at an early age to avoid getting hurt. I believed I was a failure to the core, a bum and freak that was unworthy. Mom would always tell me that I was a no good bum and would never amount to anything.

"Her hurtful words became part of me. The constant berating, cursing and physical abuse caused me to develop a defensive physical posture resulting in my having much difficulty trusting or confiding in myself or others. At an early age, I learned how to put on a façade and pretend that I was ok and learned to ignore my own needs.

"I learned not to show my emotions like to cry or that I was sad or hurt. I also developed anticipation anxiety about what was going to happen next. I had come to fear the future and frequently projected failure, death, injury, loss.

"The minute I had something to schedule I would worry: how will I get there; what will I say; will people reject me or insult me or put me down. Fear of rejection and fear of failure became part of my normal thought process.

"I projected pictures or images of a situation and imagined how to resolve a situation that did not exist yet. I was always worried about what would happen when my mother came home from work or elsewhere. Was she going to hurt me verbally or physically? I never knew what to expect.

"From my age 11 to 17, we relocated to Hallandale, Florida with both my mother and father who later rejoined the family. They got back together and me and my two brothers experienced less anger from mom as she now had some support from my father.

"Dad had PTSD from WWII and was depressed a lot and quiet when he got home from work. Mostly he would be found curled up on the couch in pain or depressed over things he wouldn't discuss. Now there was more freedom for me to leave the house and explore my new territory. I made some friends but still had deep emotional scars from those five years living with mom in Pittsburgh.

"I had low self-esteem but managed to start enjoying teenage things such as drive-in movies, dating, girlfriends, earning money to pay for some things from small jobs. I enjoyed the outdoors and socializing with a few friends.

"I enlisted in the Marine Corps at the age of 17 over forty-eight years ago but knew little about how it would change my life. My Marine Corps boot camp training at Parris Island, South Carolina was very stressful, difficult, and traumatic for me.

"The drill instructors scared all of us so I learned to keep my mouth shut, to listen, and to follow orders. There was a time I was caught talking to another marine recruit in the latrine without permission. The drill instructor became very agitated and choked me for disobeying the rules, really scaring me.

"This was the beginning of a series of deep emotional scars that left a permanent mark deep inside of me. After boot camp I went to Camp Lejeune, S.C., and later to Camp Pendleton, CA. for advanced training. This prepared me to follow orders and undergo tremendous physical and emotional stress without questioning why. In other words, I learned to do what I was told.

"I was soon to learn that there was no preparation for what I was about to experience in Vietnam. After training I was assigned to be an infantry soldier often called grunts or ground pounders. Upon arriving in Vietnam, I was assigned to a distinguished marine regiment that was later known as the Dying Nine.

"In that regiment my battalion was singled out for destruction by the enemy. Our foes called us the Walking Dead. Fortunately, I did not know at the time that the casualty rate for my unit was about 80% killed or wounded.

"I was assigned to the 1st Battalion, 9th Marines - Third Marine Division. My assignment in Vietnam in March of 1968 was at the Khe Sahn combat base around the end of the Tet offensive. This base was under frequent attack by the NVA.

Instantly I learned how to survive as I became a constant target for the enemy along with my fellow Marines. For my four months in Vietnam, I was subject to almost daily rocket and mortar attacks from the North Vietnamese Army (NVA). Much of my anxiety, fear, and hypervigilance came from trying to stay alive while dodging incoming rockets, mortars, and bullets from enemy snipers.

"Each time we were attacked there were casualties resulting in dead or wounded Marines. We rarely encountered the enemy face to face as they mostly hid from our view and fired at us from a distance.

"Many bombs exploded near me sometimes up to two to four times per day. I thought I was going to get killed almost every hour of every day while I was in Vietnam. I had become shell shocked although I had to continue to stay on the battlefield.

"On June 18, 1968, my unit was on patrol. We were resting after reaching the location we were assigned to in Quang Tri Provence. An NVA soldier appeared at the edge of the bomb crater I was in and I became startled as he was only about 30 to 40 feet from me.

"When I saw him I immediately stood up and faced him with my M16 rifle in hand. He fired his AK47 assault rifle and a bullet hit my wrist causing my M16 to drop.

"I immediately crawled to the back of the bomb crater to take protection in the high elephant grass and I crouched down waiting in fear that the enemy would find me helpless. Fortunately, another marine came to my assistance and we crawled over to a shallow depression where we found a corpsman.

"Another wounded marine and I waited there until the firefight was over. I was then transported to a first aid station in Vietnam and then transferred to Japan. Eventually I arrived at Key West Naval Hospital in July of 1968 where I was treated for a shattered wrist and gangrene.

"It took four months of mega doses of antibiotics to take care of the infection. Narcotics were administered daily to kill the pain but they didn't numb me enough to suppress the cries of pain and anguish around the clock from other wounded soldiers.

"Ultimately, I was medically and honorably discharged in February, 1969, from Jacksonville Naval Air Station with a gunshot wound and a permanently shattered wrist. Once that healed I would be fine, or so I thought.

"Over the next 40 years my mental state got progressively worse due to untreated and severe chronic combat-related PTSD. I turned off all of my emotions in combat except anger and fear with this continuing non-stop after I got out of the military.

"The daily nonstop combat survival mode I have been in all these civilian years has caused me much internal physical and emotional pain. After I got out of the USMC I finished my high school and used my GI bill benefits to complete an A.A. degree in Electronics Technology.

"Then I worked as a computer technician for 16 years and later at other technical jobs. All this time I was in denial that I had PTSD, but was aware that I had anger problems. I tried talk therapy with psychologists for much of those 40 years but that didn't bring relief to my PTSD symptoms.

"One time I went into a rage and pushed my wife saying, *'stop yelling because you are going to alert the enemy.'* During this time period I was using prescription medications off and on for pain and other symptoms. I truly believed that the many doctors I saw knew how to fix me.

"Eventually in 2009 the emotional and physical stress elevated to a point where I was having daily panic attacks, homicidal and suicidal ideations, hyper-vigilance, rages, startle response, foreshortened future fears, nightmares, depression and anxiety. I also had chronic neck and low back pain and difficulty with routine everyday activities of daily living.

"Fortunately, I was finally and correctly diagnosed with chronic combat related PTSD and was determined to be disabled. I spent the next two years going through the VA system finally attaining a permanent and total disability rating.

"In order to do this, I had to obtain the assistance of outside civilian doctors to support my claim. Unfortunately, over the last 40 years, traditional treatment such as drug medications and talk therapy have not helped my PTSD symptoms.

"When I first got out of the USMC it seemed as if I was ok for the first seven years. Eventually I started self-medicating with alcohol and drugs. After a while I switched addictions to food, specifically focusing obsessively on sugar and carbs. Eventually I became bulimic, purging with laxatives.

"I have been in a 12-step recovery for bulimia and compulsive overeating for the past 14 years. I have been able to become abstinent from the addiction of my trigger foods and overeating over the past few years and continue to attend 12 step meeting as my primary source of help for my bulimic condition.

"I recently had some improvement with childhood issues by doing forgiveness work on myself and my mother. The gunshot wound to my left wrist caused my body to be stuck in a defensive posture - a pattern that has remained for over 40 years.

"Looking at me from the outside I appear normal physically. However, the entire left side of my body and my left arm and leg has neuropathy. My left side has about half the strength as my right side resulting in fatigue after activity. My current diagnoses are anemia and chronic adrenal fatigue.

"Regarding my anger, I find that it happens when I'm in the kitchen doing food preparation and my wife and I are arguing. This happens when she disagrees and I feel she does not support me. I find that when we both argue our viewpoints and neither is willing to compromise, I get triggered.

"When this happens, I need to go out somewhere, like I had to escape from the house when I was a child and then come back home to the site of the trauma. I'm afraid that if I refuse my wife's request to do something she wants, she will be angry and yell at me. I am afraid when I have to leave the house to go on a routine errand or appointment I will not return alive.

"I'm afraid thinking that I may die like in Vietnam prior to going out on another deadly patrol. The company commander would shout out: *OK men, 'Saddle up! – I thought, I'm going out again on another suicide patrol not knowing if I will return alive. I always thought I would get killed or wounded, just didn't know when.'"*

'Alice's Story'

"I met Paul in 1975 at a college in Pennsylvania. He was a letter carrier at a local post office and appeared to be someone that had plans for a better future, like myself. He was studying for an electronics degree in order to eventually secure a better paying career in computer repair.

"He seemed a little shy at first, but he was nice and I thought that he was cute. We started dating and we did a lot of different things like going on trips to New York or New England as well as attending concerts, dinner, etc. We had fun together and started living together after finding an apartment near my parent's home in Pennsylvania.

"Once this occurred, things changed. There was a lot of arguing and fighting about how Paul thought I should do things like cleaning and other household activities. As we furthered in our careers, the romance diminished as Paul's anger got worse and worse.

"Eventually he became violent: throwing and breaking furniture; throwing food; becoming verbally and physically abusive to me. At times, he would go into rages and I was afraid for my life. He hurt me on occasions, injuring me both physically and emotionally. I told him he needed help but he didn't think he did.

"He voluntarily enrolled in a domestic violence course and that didn't help. Paul still gets angry but not always with that intensity. His rages are not as frequent but are spontaneous and without warning.

"He seems aloof at times, like he doesn't care about me and is consumed with himself and his eating program as well as the people in his program. Sometimes if I say or do something he doesn't agree with, he gets angry and storms out of the room, abandoning me. When that occurs, I feel helpless and upset.

"If I speak while he is talking, he'll either abruptly leave the room or humiliates me, even in front of others. It seems like everything has to be about him and his life. He goes out of his way calling it service by treating others with more concern than me, often talking for hours trying to help them. But he treats me differently, like he doesn't love me anymore.

"If I disagree with something he is trying to get across, he raises his voice and yells and talks down to me and keeps repeating it over and over loudly. He can't seem to discuss differences of opinion in any other way. This is a continual problem with him. He doesn't share anything with me separating things he does from me. I feel like I'm not a part of his life anymore. He often seems miserable, whether it's his health or seemingly always waking up on the wrong side of the bed.

"If I ask him if he could do something for me, he often refuses and argues that he will not be told or asked to do anything by me. He is also very serious, controlling, and doesn't smile or laugh much. He doesn't seem to know how to have fun anymore. He often uses ear plugs and says, I'm talking too loudly, and then he proceeds to ignore me. "

As a prelude to the next chapter, I'll share Paul's overview of his RESET Therapy experience. He notes that: "After many years of traditional therapy for my PTSD related symptoms and conditions which included psychotropic medicines and talk therapy for anger, depression, homicidal and suicidal ideations, foreshortened future, hyper vigilance, dissociation, projecting death right around the corner, I finally found a therapy that works.

I now have a sense of peace and well-being I never had previously. I feel better able to cope with everyday routine problems and life issues without constant anxiety and panic attacks. I also found a way to resolve the deep depression that has been with me since Vietnam in 1968. I use both logic and emotion more routinely and can think more quickly. I come up with ideas and express myself more spontaneously.

"Reset Therapy has reduced my anxiety and anger. I don't remember when I ever felt this way. My fight or flight switch is turned off and I do not feel the constant adrenalin/cortisol rush from anxiety and fear. I am better able to focus on a single task without intrusive thoughts and dissociation: something that was very prevalent on a daily basis. I feel more relaxed and am able to make decisions based on what is best for me instead of people pleasing.

"I can and do use RESET whenever I choose, instead of picking up my addiction to soothe the pain and suffering when difficult situations arise. The addictive response to my problems only causes me and those close to me more trouble and pain.

"I am in the process of deprogramming from the part of my Marine Corps training that is harmful to me in my everyday life. I now know I am not a constant danger to myself and others due to my explosive rage that has been with me all these years.

"In fact, it's significantly diminished! I have a better relationship with my wife and with myself. I sleep better and am not constantly problem solving and obsessing about what to do and how to do it. I am very grateful for this life saving therapy. Dr. George has been a wonderful mentor and coach through this process. His guidance and support has been the key to my success.

Thank you Dr. George!"

Chapter Eight:

'Fidelity, Honor, Valor'

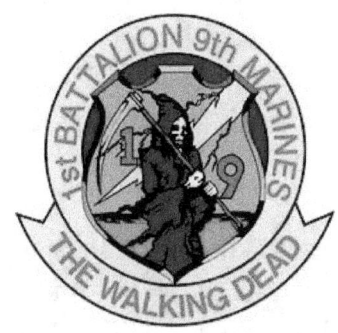

The following e-mail notes were selected in order to share with you the unfolding process that Paul experienced, sometimes on a day to day basis. I have edited out more than half of the correspondence due to the excessive length of the material. I have kept progress notes that display Paul's emerging awareness of his status as well as the positive steps he has taken to function in a world he has previously been a stranger to.

I have not significantly changed the substance of his or Alice's correspondence to me. Alice's input will be italicized. My specific e-mail replies to Paul are underlined to provide you with my reactions, directives, etc., in reply to his progress notes. At first,

Paul responded on an almost daily basis revealing his strong need and desire for guidance and acceptance.

Interesting, the distance and lack of personal intimacy that is typically developed within the face to face therapeutic experience likely permitted him to truly develop a deep and full relationship with me. In retrospect, this seemed to be a good alternative to his going through a difficult transference relationship to get to a point of mutual trust.

Meaningful aspects of his correspondence are included so that you might be an inside observer to the hurdles Paul faced. In addition, you share the tremendous courage he evidenced in pushing through a life time of barriers that blocked him from fully transformed into the person he became capable of being.

Paul - 3/05/14 "The unit was delivered this afternoon. I left it on the table having to run some errands and having a stressful day. On a scale of 1-10, by that evening I was at a 10 with rage, anger and homicidal thoughts flowing through my mind. By that time, I got home, hungry, angry and pissed off, I decided to wait to eat dinner and use RESET, even though I wanted to eat which made me even angrier.

"I used the same settings Dr. George found for me when we met and let all of the feelings flow into the sound. The first five to ten minutes, I allowed the feelings within me to surface and saw flashes of anger and fear with my mother, boot camp, Vietnam.

"Then the last ten minutes or so, the anger and rages and everything subsided and all I could see, hear or feel was the annoying buzzing of the sound. After the treatment, I sat next to Alice at the computer, helping her while she ordered an item online. I worked with her with patience and kindness; something I rarely did especially in the evening, my worst time with PTSD. On a scale of 1-10, I felt like I was a zero, quite amazing!"

"Paul, it looks like your setting is good for the anxiety targets. Let me suggest that you use RESET selectively now when the strong feelings come up, particularly with the PTSD triggers.

"I'm thinking that our e-mail correspondence is a good way to capture your response to this intervention because it will provide me with an in-the-moment source of clarity. I wonder if Alice would be willing to keep me posted regarding how she's seeing you change through e-mail as well?"

Paul - 3/7/14 – "I woke up with typical fears like I need women to protect me and looking for my sister to protect me. Later in the afternoon, after a nap, I was in a foul mood and argued with Alice about doing some tasks I expected her to do. I started having the same feeling towards her that I had toward mom for locking me up in the basement tied to the boiler and left all alone.

"Mom would try to restrict me from leaving the house and I hated her for it. I did a treatment with my anger level about an 8 with it going to 1 to 2 when done. I also had back pain at a 7 level on the 10-point pain scale. After treatment, my back pain was about a 1. Afterwards, I felt good for the rest of the evening."

Paul - 3/11/14 "I'm starting to notice that I am more animated in my interactions. Yesterday I was at a 12-step group meeting and interacting with three other people, doing recovery based learning. I was surprised that I was able to pick up and learn concepts without confusion. I was relating stories about my aunts and uncles and one of the women said, 'I detect a Pittsburgh accent.'

"I was surprised that I was relaxed enough to recognize that some of the people there did care about me and paid attention to me. I was in my car taking a nap and they went looking for me. I fell asleep and went into the meeting late and was surprised that people really did like me and were concerned for my safety."

Paul - 3/12/14 "Interesting day – woke up and did a treatment right away. I noticed a pattern of awakening with the traumatic memories and accompanying thought processes. It feels like someone is looking to get at me to kill me or try to harm me. Survival mode thinking still seems normal to me. Not every day is like this but now that I am doing these treatments there is a change in my intensity level."

Paul - 3/13/14 "I notice that when I'm tired and fatigued, PTSD symptoms start to come back. I ate lunch and went to sleep for about two hours and woke up in a very scary but familiar mode different than this morning. It was a full fight or flight response.

"We had an appointment to see the landscape lady and I was anxious. Alice asked me some questions and I was abrupt and said leave me alone for ½ hour while you drive to the landscape place. I did a treatment in the car and wow, it turned out to be mostly about Viet Nam.

"It was when I was terrified about going out on patrols and not knowing if we were going to die that moment or not. I was able to eventually feel accepting of my traumatic experience and by the time we arrived at the landscape nursery, I was ok.

"I was able to work with the landscaper and agree on the specifics of the design. I was also aware of how unusually friendly she was to both Alice and I. These good feelings lasted the rest of the day and I did not react to Alice's comments.

"I think as a child that I was so broken that I erased myself as a person at about age 7 in order to deal with the abuse and brutality related to living with my mother. I became a non-entity and as I grew older I took on the personality of people I admired like John Wayne or other male actors like William Holden. Tough guys.

"Now that I desire to be grounded in the present, I find my mind always drifting to these faces outside my house. I realize that my belief system is based on my thought that it will be better outside.

"I think that RESET has been reducing my PTSD and now my brain is able to understand and learn new concepts, unlike my survival brain on PTSD. So now I am having to differentiate between true PTSD anxiety (fight or flight) vs. anxiety based on irrational thoughts and unrealistic expectations."

Alice – "While Paul was talking to his sponsor Jim on the speaker phone, Jim made a negative comment about me. I felt bad because I thought he and his wife were our friends. Paul agreed with me that it was not appropriate for Jim to comment about me that way. Paul showed me support and care. This is unusual for Paul to stick up for me."

Paul - 3/14/14 – "I have identified two core issues that are of importance to me. With the first: I have to get out of my house in order to feel and be safe. With the second: I need to have people validate me as being ok, real, worthy and loved. I woke up this morning anxious, thinking I can't wait to leave the house so I can see people.

"I also see visions of people's faces from the last few days or those of people I will be seeing. That may be from thinking I am not alive as a child and need to see people to figure out who I am supposed to be today."

Alice – *"This morning Paul seemed peaceful and nice. I wasn't around him most of the day. In the early evening, we ran some errands and he seemed okay until I verbalized about writing and thinking back and he became agitated and nasty, his normal self. I asked him should you be using RESET and he said no because he was disagreeing with me about something, not sure what."*

"Alice, I'm going to advise you to refrain from suggesting to Paul that he needs RESET. I know that you want to help him but, if you suggest treatment to him at a particular time, he will increasingly see you as behaving like his mother. When he is dealing with difficult material it is best that you be a safe and warm cushion for him to cling to. In this way, you become his beloved wife rather than his despised mother."

Paul - 3/16/14 "This morning I focused on and fully experienced the fear as you advised. I targeted the feelings in my shoulders and neck and felt it in my body. Eventually thoughts and images arose of the DI in boot camp saying don't look at me and don't talk unless you're given permission.

"I did my best to feel and become part of that experience. When it diminished, the next image was of my mother expressing that I should not be seen or heard and to shut up. I went into that experience as fully as I could, seeing it and feeling the fear all over my upper body.

"At first it was difficult not to run from it but I decided not to rush it and to take my time. Eventually I found myself verbalizing it saying out loud, 'I can't talk or you may kill me.' It may have been from childhood or Vietnam or both.

"Verbalizing it helped me to clarify the specific fear. I noted the settings for future use and noted that today's session was longer than previous ones lasting about 25 minutes. Later in the morning, I noticed some other trauma issues and noted them for my next session."

"Paul, I'm following your notes closely and notice that objectivity is beginning to evidence itself in your reports. This confirms for me that you're really putting yourself fully into the process. Thus, I'd like to take you to the next level in your exploration using RESET Therapy.

You will be finding that there are different brain circuits that we are targeting through your focusing on them. The first of course is that the anxiety protocol is primarily triggered through fear and anxiety. In essence, you are to become the fear/anxiety throughout the 15/20 minutes of treatment. This is frightening but it is the path to take to fully free you from this aspect of your complex PTSD. Thus, rather than running from the house, you are to stay there & nuke the fear!"

Paul - 3-21-14 "This was a great opportunity for me to use RESET Therapy. I overate last night and felt guilty and fearful about going to my 12-step meeting this morning. I started in my old thinking mode of imagining people at the meeting rejecting or hurting me or belittling me like mom did.

"At first I was afraid to admit mistakes to mom and eventually came to accept that she had a right to discipline me even if I did not like it. This acknowledgement let me move from my usual state of fear to a new one of acceptance.

"I am much more understanding and caring now about Alice's feelings and believe there is more of a positive emotional connection between us. I can feel a bond starting to form. I also feel compassion and love for her, even though I don't always agree with her."

"Paul, you'll notice that as the trauma poison leaves you, other targets will surface almost in a cue like fashion. After a while, your mind will put them in the hopper instinctively. As you come to trust in the process, the core aspects of who you truly are will solidify. You're doing well with becoming more specific with RESET Therapy tuning. As the anxiety/fear diminishes, so will the level of anger."

Alice - 3-29-14 *"Paul seems to be a lot calmer after using RESET. However, at times he has the same issues with me going in the kitchen while he is concentrating with his food preparations. He still acts the same at times; i.e. stressed, angry, mean, pushy, arrogant, and impatient.*

"We still do not spend a lot of time together as we spend about 8 hours a day each day with house issues plus he has meetings, phone calls, appointments, etc. It is my opinion that he needs to use RESET more frequently so that he can be calmer throughout the day on a daily basis, rather than for only one issue at a particular time."

Paul - 4/03/14 "I am changing my attitudes and belief system toward a more positive one. Now, I only use RESET when it is needed. I know that it really works and I'm getting a better awareness and feel for when to use it. The first problem I recognize is my tendency to deny that I have a problem to myself.

"After I admit that I am anxious, I have come to trust that the treatment will help. It really takes time for me to trust anything. It's like peeling off onion layers. When I address a current situation, it seems to connect with and clear up the original cause from the past. Then the next day something that was deeply suppressed in my mind comes up."

"Paul, I'd like to discuss one of your core difficulties which is: 'I have to get out of my house in order to feel and be safe.' Now I believe that your progress suggests that it is time to take this one on. To do it, you must face the fear head-on by staying in the house till it is resolved. Of course, use the RESET-Anxiety setting for this one.

Keep me appraised of how this one is going through telephone contact if necessary. The worst will come once and then it will fade and be fully gone from you. Only in this way can you truly be free of it. Through this scary process, you will come to feel the confidence in yourself that you so desperately seek from others. Paul, this is the path that you have come to trust. Now push it to the max marine."

Paul - 4/09/14 "As soon as I saw your e-mail, I took a different approach to RESET. Rather than going into my bedroom to do a RESET intervention, I stayed out in the common living areas and decided to do RESET when I felt the need.

"On Saturday I had a lot of success with doing just what you suggested. I did a RESET without limiting the time I needed to completely resolve the ongoing delusion/flashback. I had very positive results so far, this weekend with the new concept. I can stay right here and face whatever it is, right in the middle of my real area of stress. I can be around live people starting with Alice. I appreciate your support and will call if I need to."

Paul - 4/20/14 "I discovered one of my core issues is that since I was about 6 or 7 years old, I rejected my family of origin and have been searching for another family that is kind and loving and joyful. I remember taking walks and imagining how nice it would be to be in another person's home. All throughout the years when I was in another person's home I felt safe and secure.

"Also, a significant part of RESET is helping me clear out the trauma from the brutal treatment I received in the Marine Corps boot camp. The deadly philosophy that I've applied in the real world was that as marines we never stop or give up until our enemy is overcome and defeated.

"I previously looked at people as being the friendlies or the enemy which was for me a very sick and harmful way to approach life. Some of my RESET situations related to my going out on suicide operations called search and destroy missions.

"I have come to believe that the enemy (NVA) was mostly destroyed by our US air support and we the ground soldiers were used as bait to get the enemy soldiers out of hiding. I realize today it is a blessing that I made it out of there alive."

Paul - 6-21-15 "After a reset session a week or so ago I had some clarity regarding my relationship with Alice. When I was between the ages of 6 and 9 my trauma at home was so difficult I erased myself from living and feeling.

"I killed Paul off to save him from mom's abuse. I also eventually turned off all my emotions and feelings toward her in my home in Pittsburgh. My relationship with myself and mother was false. Neither she nor I really existed in my mind, that's the only way I could cope with her abuse.

"I brought the same beliefs into my marriage. I ignored Alice when she wanted my attention. I almost always say no - no - no immediately to almost any request she may have made of me. This is why Alice feels like our relationship is doomed.

"If I don't exist and neither does she, no progress will ever be made. As she has said, 'Paul seems totally ok with other people outside of our home.' It is true. I can open up and have a meaningful relationship with people outside my home.

"Therapy has helped me in that respect, I work beautifully with others but not with the person I'm supposed to love. How could I if she does not exist to me as a real person? I am finally becoming aware of my dilemma and my blinders."

"Paul, insight is beginning to be present in your comments. This is clearly a sign that you are breaking through the instinctive survival reactions and using more advanced processing abilities to figure out what is triggering you. You are reaching your goal."

I end the comments and responses here as you are certainly aware by now that this is an ongoing therapeutic process. This becomes a much more traditional therapy interchange than the quick results reported in non-complex PTSD cases.

Hopefully you've also noticed that Paul is now firmly in the world of reality rather than in the delusional mode he was previously in. He is rebuilding his sense of self-esteem, brick by brick, issue by issue. I believe that his addictive difficulties have been stabilized, his marriage has a chance and his hope for the future finally has a firm foundation.

I continue to follow Paul although he rarely needs advice or support at this point in time. I consider this to be the best type of compliment I could possibly receive!

Epilogue:

In the face of an onslaught of increasing need related to the effects of trauma, a recent analysis (May, 2015) of 70 Cognitive Behavioral Therapy studies that were done between 1977 and 2014 has raised some eyebrows. The authors (Johnsen, T. J., & Friborg, O.) concluded that Cognitive Behavioral Therapy (CBT) is roughly half as effective in treating depression as it was previously thought to be.

"CBT has had hundreds if not thousands of studies performed evaluating its effectiveness and it has become the 'workhorse' and most accepted model of emotional and psychological psychotherapeutic intervention, accepted ubiquitously in institutions and for insurance reimbursement."

To further compound the above CBT findings, Jay C. Fournier, MA, et. al., published a paper in the Journal of the American Medical Association (2010) entitled: Antidepressant Drug Effects and Depression Severity: A Patient-Level Meta-analysis. Note was made that:

"Antidepressant medications represent the best-established treatment for major depressive disorder, but there is little evidence that they have a specific pharmacological effect relative to pill placebo for patients with less severe depression." The objective of the study was to measure medication benefits as compared to placebo "across a wide range of initial symptom severity in patients diagnosed with depression."

My interpretation of the above two findings is that the mainstream intervention for treating PTSD with accompanying depression is showing flaws in its original promise. This vital information is emerging within the context of the general public becoming far more aware and concerned about the development of effective interventions for large numbers of PTSD and depression affected veterans.

To repeat, as noted in the first of the above two articles, a previously publicized mainstream therapy (CBT) is not holding up to the rigorous research that is now available for analysis of reported results. In addition, there is the issue of provider resources. There is little question that current therapy options require intensive time with limited numbers of professionally trained individuals available.

The second article relates to the use of the 'pill' as the panacea for treating the emotional component of the PTSD and depression condition. The comparative analysis in this case finds no difference in other than severe depression conditions. Thus, the two mainstream interventions touted as the solution for trauma sufferer's falls apart in the light of modern analysis.

We are all too aware of the emotional impact from the 9/11 World Trade Center disaster as well as the deaths and injuries resulting from varied wars this country has been involved in. Add to this the natural disasters like Hurricane Katrina as well as worldwide traumatic events such as the Asian tsunami and other large-scale unforeseen events.

The increasing number of people being traumatized throughout the world on a daily basis demands that we do something about their circumstances. The 22 veterans who choose suicide on a daily basis require us to do something about their plight!

In my practice as earlier described, I have seen amazing changes that occurred in a short period of time with complete remission forthcoming from RESET Therapy. This finding is also reported by numerous colleagues also using neuromodulation procedures with their patients.

The primary question then becomes one of how to effect change in a system of care that is currently largely ineffective in addressing a problem that is a major issue in our society. The answer is before us if we are willing to approach this challenge in an innovative and open minded manner.

Over the past several years, I have been on a one-person mission attempting to share my findings with national decision makers, senators, VA representatives and the therapeutic community at large, to little or no avail. I have not yet been able to find my way through bureaucratic hurdles to bring this break-through treatment to public awareness.

RESET Therapy offers a new paradigm: a neural model vs. talk therapy. As for me, I cannot let this rest. Even though I am technically retired at 75 years of age, I am in the planning stages for a formal fMRI study to further document cortical changes forthcoming from the RESET Therapy treatment intervention.

My hope is that this will stimulate further studies, and in time, produce acceptance and widespread use of this new intervention. I view the first fMRI study as equivalent to the laying of the cornerstone in a new structure. From this will come formal scientific studies using matched comparison groups.

As I discussed earlier, I am committed to getting the word out about RESET Therapy and have chosen the online print option through Kindle as a beginning point rather than waiting years to publish through traditional channels. With 22 of our veterans taking their own lives on a daily basis, we can ill afford to delay advances in treating this terrible problem one day longer than necessary.

Detail will be provided regarding sequential books to be made available. A companion book to this text specifically designed for 'healers' is in the draft stage now. This new text is targeted to those who treat victims of trauma as well as their families in order to hasten the end of unnecessary suffering.

As this awareness spreads, it is my goal to prepare healers to utilize RESET Therapy for transformative purposes. I invite you to join me on this journey, first through your participation and involvement in my LinkedIn group (RESET Therapy), which welcomes both healers, those who continue to experience the effects of PTSD and family members. Next, follow my sequential books covering corollary topics such as: depression, unresolved grief/survivor's guilt, addiction, chronic pain and complex PTSD.

I intend to add a book focusing on our heroic first responders such as the police, fire fighters, ambulance drivers, etc. who face the potential impact of trauma each and every time they report to work. Finally, since Traumatic Brain Injury (TBI) is such a signature component for so many of our returning veterans, I intend to recruit my fellow professionals willing to help me to explore whether RESET

Therapy may assist those injured by concussion or other form of head injury.

From the cornerstone of the first fMRI case study of a PTSD volunteer that is yet to happen, let us together look forward to a completed structure deserving of those who served and sacrificed, but remain unhealed. It is to my fellow veterans that I dedicate my commitment to pursue this goal for as long as I am able to do so.

Final Bit of Sharing:

In the book you've just completed, you've read of Shawn. He's also to be in this next book, but guess what? I don't want to leave your hanging so I'm including this as sort of an invite to read the next one that's coming.

As Shawn reports: "On my third and final visit with Doctor Lindenfeld, he asked me how things were going and I told him that I only had one episode of night sweats. At first, I didn't think that there was anything wrong but he suggested that we do a slightly different kind of treatment with the sound that he called a 'disappointment/ worry/ depression protocol'. I thought long and hard and the only thing I could come up with that was still bothering me was my brother.

"I mentally reviewed the timeline of my life thinking about my youth and my relationship with my brother while listening to the sound. I couldn't believe it but all of a sudden, I felt like a tidal wave of emotion came over me and I burst into continuous tears and sobbing.

"All I could say during that explosion of emotions was, 'he was my brother and he was supposed to protect me.' After that release, I felt like the weight of the world had come off my shoulders.

"In retrospect, my brother and I dealt differently with not knowing our father. I couldn't miss someone I never knew. My brother idealized him and couldn't seem to get away from the loss. I grew up never getting in trouble and always trying to do what was right.

"My brother is presently serving 12 years in prison for attempted murder. He's been in and out of prison since he was 18 and he is presently 44 years old. I have not spoken to him in over 25 years. I've come to forgive him and feel sorry for him.

"After that last session, I felt exhausted. I felt like every ounce of energy had been sucked from my body. I drove home, talked to my wife a little bit and went to bed because I was so tired.

"The next morning, I awoke with a profound sense of being a new man. Since the last treatment, I've come to enjoy life, no more cold sweats, sleepless nights or being an 'ass-hole.' The three things that I'm so happy about are that I'm smiling again, I'm laughing again and I found joy in my life."